MOKITA

How to navigate PERIMENOPAUSE with confidence & ease

Featuring 13 Women's Health Professionals

SHIRLEY WEIR

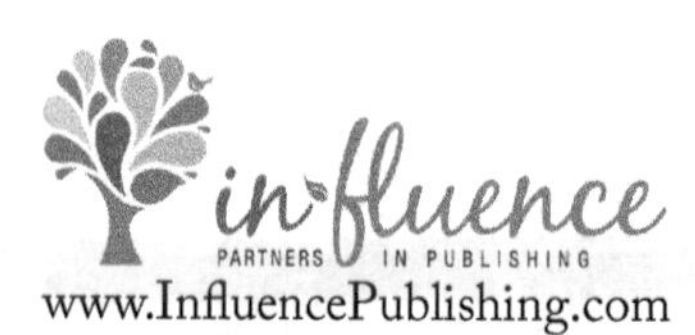

www.InfluencePublishing.com

Published by Menopause Chicks, October 2018
ISBN: 9781999470104

Editor: Danielle Anderson
Typeset: Greg Salisbury
Book Cover Design: Judith Mazari

Disclaimer: The content of this book is for informational purposes only and is not intended to be a substitute for professional medical advice or treatment advice of any kind. Menopause Chicks does not provide medical advice, diagnosis or treatment. Always consult a physician or other qualified health provider before starting any new treatment or protocol, or with any questions you may have regarding perimenopause, menopause or other health-related experience.

This book is dedicated to an extraordinary woman I am proud to call my BFF and my sister. **Brenda**, you were your own best health advocate long before I even knew what that phrase meant. Thank you for being my lighthouse for my entire life. I love you to the moon and back. xo

~

This book is dedicated to my friend, **Dr. Sue Buchan**. Sue, there ought to be a picture of you beside the word "care" in the dictionary, because that is what you do best. I know family physicians have one of the most challenging jobs on this planet, and you fulfill your role with grace. I have watched you share your genius and your heart with your family, your friends, and your community. I will be forever inspired. xo

~

This book is dedicated to **YOU**. The ultimate goal on this journey is to feel healthy and vibrant and to have the energy to do the things we want to do. The transition through perimenopause to menopause can be seamless, or it can be a struggle, or it can be somewhere in between. There are, unfortunately, no predictors for how it will be for you. However, one thing you can be certain of, and take charge of, is being your own best health advocate. Regardless of your age right now, I invite you to get as informed as you possibly can. Be prepared and commit to doing a little (or a lot) of work in order to find the journey and support you need and desire.

I beg you to know this, and to believe it with all your heart:

You are worth it.

And, you are not alone.

Thank you for putting your own name at the top of the to-do list.

xo

"We delight in the beauty of the **butterfly**, but rarely admit the changes it has gone through to achieve that beauty."

– Maya Angelou

Table of Contents

Author's Note

This book is an introduction to perimenopause. It is not an all-inclusive guide or a substitute for you doing your own research, speaking with your own health care team, and making decisions about your midlife health that are right for you.

This book is a great place to begin your own learning, or to clarify your knowledge; to check on the accuracy of what you know, or think you know, about navigating perimenopause. It will be especially helpful if you don't have time to read thirty books or spend hundreds of hours scouring the internet, trying to figure out what information is reliable and what is trash—there is plenty of both. The ultimate goal of this book is to make you feel less alone as you journey through this new life phase.

This book is not a magic wand. In fact, I prefer to tell women that navigating perimenopause and midlife health is more like solving a Rubik's cube, where the goal is for you to complete one side at a time. Did you know the centre piece of a Rubik's cube never moves? Let's pretend that centre piece is you, and all the other pieces are moving around you to conform to your best possible health. That's right—you are at the core of your midlife health journey. All the pieces around you include information and education, health care professionals, relationships, self-talk, attitude, and your decisions about how you are going to eat, move, sleep and manage stress. The more informed and empowered you become, the easier it will be to align all the colours on all sides of your cube.

To assist in solving your midlife health puzzle, I invited thirteen incredible women's health professionals to join me on this project, including an acupuncturist, a cannabis advocate, a chiropractor, a dietitian, a doctor of natural medicine, a doctor of naturopathic medicine, an energy healer, a hormone expert, a meditation coach, a personal coach, a pharmacist, a physician, and a vagina coach/pelvic health expert. I am so grateful they all jumped at the opportunity to contribute to this project so we can empower more women, like you, to build their own integrated health team.

Their chapters offer insights into the benefits of working with each modality, and help save you time and the stress of not knowing if one particular journey resonates with you. You may even see yourself in some of the examples shared.

For the most part, the stories in this book deal with natural menopause. Many women in our Private Online Community (Facebook.com/groups/MenopauseChicks) are also dealing with a broad range of other conditions, including surgical menopause (via partial or full hysterectomies), premenstrual dysphoric disorder, endometriosis, and more. I want you to know we see you too, and we honour you, as you often serve as our role models for what it means to be our own best health advocates.

We hope this book either confirms your knowledge or brings a new or fresh perspective to how all of us view, think about, or talk about perimenopause and menopause—especially if you've ever (consciously or unconsciously) equated menopause with negativity. It might prompt you to consider how you approach your next conversation about menopause, be it with a health professional, your partner or spouse, a co-worker, your family, or your children. It could prompt you to change the way you take in messages about menopause from experts, the media, advertisers, or casual conversations.

This book is not me saying, "Hey, look over here—I have all the answers!" As a midlife woman, and as a women's health advocate, I have been researching this topic for the better part of the last twelve years, and I don't believe anyone has all the answers. However, I do think that women have the right to awesome information, that we deserve to have a great quality of life, and that at this stage of our lives, we may need guidance in order to navigate perimenopause with confidence and ease.

I hope this book is helpful to you, and to those who love you.

Introduction: MOKITA

Mokita is a word from the Kivila language spoken on the largest of the Trobriand Islands, just off the coast of Papua New Guinea. Translated, it means "a truth we all know, and agree not to talk about." In North America, we often refer to this as "the elephant in the room."

Perimenopause and menopause are excellent examples of mokitas, although I would argue that most times they aren't even allowed in the room! They are treated like some creepy or questionable stranger who lurks outside the window while everyone pretends not to see it, or know it, assuming that ignoring it means it will somehow just go away.

I have been fascinated by the word mokita for some time now. Back in 2012, when I launched MenopauseChicks.com with the tagline "Cracking Open the Conversation," I naively thought that it was a lack of conversation that was the problem. I assumed that all we had to do was bring menopause out of the closet, and then we could magically eradicate all the confusing and conflicting information on women's midlife health.

It turns out I was only partially right. What I quickly discovered when I stood up and announced I was a *perimenopause chick* was that some women would push back and declare they were not yet ready to talk about, or learn about, perimenopause and menopause. I was surprised to encounter this, and I was curious to find out why there was such resistance to having conversations about menopause.

So, why do we not talk about mokitas? How did some topics—such as reproductive health, hormone health, sexual health, money, relationships, and mental and emotional health—not earn a seat at the table or around the water cooler? Why is it socially acceptable to say "I went to the dentist this morning" but, uncouth to say "I went for a Pap smear"? It could be that we are afraid of the reaction we might get; it could also be that we fear being judged, especially in certain social settings.

Since discovering the word mokita, I have also heard it referred to as "polite fiction." This is where everyone is generally aware of a particular truth but pretends to believe some alternative version, sometimes to avoid shame or embarrassment. Challenging these polite fictions, I've learned, can conjure up resistance.

I am really not one who likes to talk about bodily functions. However, I had a strong compulsion to ensure women were more informed and felt less alone on their journey. I had also watched and read enough Brené Brown to know that if I truly wanted to make a shift in the menopause/women's health movement, I would need to allow myself to be vulnerable. So, I started saying the word menopause at cocktail parties and backyard BBQs and boardroom tables. I said it to men, women, and young teens. I said it to friends, business associates, and neighbours. There were some slow nods, a few blank stares, some uncomfortable giggles, and plenty of awkward silences, all of which added up to some unexpected pushback. Friends said, "I didn't know you were fifty yet" (I was forty-six at the time)—as if fifty is the only socially acceptable age for a woman to begin her midlife health education! (I was forty-six at the time.) It was as if fifty is the only socially acceptable age for a woman to begin her midlife health education! One woman even told me she would never discuss menopause with her physician because he was too good looking!

Thankfully, I also received many positive reactions as well. Some were very encouraging, telling me how the menopause conversation was badly needed because they either didn't have much knowledge, or they found most information to be confusing or overwhelming. Many women appeared eager to learn—whether that was by actively sharing their own stories, or passively sliding into the back row at my events and learning as much as they could via other women's questions.

In Papua New Guinea, the health of a community is actually measured by the number of mokitas; the more mokitas there are, the worse the health of the tribe will be. Knowing that mokitas can do a lot of damage if not addressed, tribal leaders reach out and address the uncomfortable truths in order to improve the health of their people.

Think about some of the generational myths we are potentially passing onto our daughters and future generations by not addressing mokitas now. Think of how effectively and efficiently we could address the questions and concerns women have about their midlife health if we had open and honest conversations around the topic. Think about how we will push OUR TRIBE to new heights as we address the mokita of menopause.

Think about how much healthier our community will be.

~

I never intended to grow up and be a *Menopause Chick.*

When I was in third year of university, I remember a group of fourth-year students surveying our class on what our ideal career of choice was. My answer was easy: I was going to be head of marketing for Coca-Cola. At the time, I was in love with their product, their ads, and the values they portrayed through their advertising. I wanted to teach the world to sing in perfect harmony. Secretly (or perhaps, thanks to social media, not so secretly), I still do.

At the age of twenty, I would have never imagined saying: "I want to grow up and be a *Menopause Chick.*" I knew absolutely nothing about menopause. No one had ever had a conversation with me about it. I did not discuss anything about my period with anyone. I cringed if someone ever said "bowel movement" in my presence. I would never say bleeding, flow, or menstruation. Talking about bodily functions gave me the heebie-jeebies.

And now, some thirty years later, I shock myself whenever I introduce myself as a *Menopause Chick.* I almost always feel as if I must add qualifiers to that title, such as "I don't have any medical expertise" and "I'm not a health expert." Early on, I played small and explained to people that I am "just" a curator of information.

WAIT, STOP RIGHT THERE. This is what my husband likes to call an "Etch-a-Sketch" moment. This is one of those times where we have to take what we are thinking and saying, turn it upside-down, and give it a shake. It is time for a paradigm shift.

Let me explain.

Menopause is not a medical condition, so why do I mention my lack of medical expertise? And as for being a health expert, who is that if it's NOT me? I am a health expert...of my own body! I am a health advocate...for myself! And you are too—or, you certainly can be. In fact, I strongly encourage you to be.

Consider puberty for a moment. Many of us have raised kids successfully through adolescence. When they had questions about the changes happening in their bodies, you may have turned to a network of available information for support. But, I can guarantee that you did not say, "Whoa, sorry honey, I'm not a medical expert." That's because puberty is a normal life phase.

So is perimenopause and menopause.

And yet, the mere mention of the word menopause can shut down the conversation in seconds flat. People do not know what to think, what to say, or how to react; many look truly dumbfounded. It's as if they immediately have images flash across their internal screens that say "Wow, she's old!" or "If she is going to talk about periods and hot flashes, I'm outta here!" On the other hand, I've also met plenty of women—and men—who want to share their stories and welcome any and all information to help smooth their journey.

In 2016, I surveyed 1000 women aged thirty-nine to fifty-five, and 70% said they didn't have anyone to talk to about menopause, OR that they would never talk about menopause with anyone! This concerned me greatly and led me to launch the Menopause Chicks Private Community on Facebook—a social learning group created to empower women to navigate perimenopause with confidence and ease. Inside the community, we answer women's questions, connect them to trustworthy information, recommend women's health professionals who can support their journey, and (the best of all) we connect women to other women for peer support and to share experiences.

Perimenopause and menopause are two of the most natural transitions in life; yet, they are also the most taboo and misunderstood.

In "A historical perspective on menopause and menopausal age" (Singh, Kaur, Walia, 2002), the authors state that the first known references to menopause can be traced back to Aristotle. A French physician coined the term menopause in 1821, and medical interest increased significantly in the 19th century. In the 1930s, people described menopause as a deficiency disease, and as a result various therapies were invented to treat it. Pharmaceuticals entered into the scenario in a big way and began to dominate the discussion. The medicalization of menopause continued to increase in the 1970s, 1980s, and 1990s. Various countries formed menopause societies to promote education and research amongst health care professionals. The use of hormone therapies sky-rocketed in western countries, where women and the medical community tended to only view menopause through a negative lens, as compared to some other cultures, such as those in India and Asia, where aging is viewed with a much more positive and respected outlook.

So, this is what we are up against: decades of menopause being thought of as a disease, a deficiency, and battling a culture that predominantly views the midlife transition as something that requires medicalization.

This also explains why vast numbers of women feel uninformed about what to expect in perimenopause and menopause. We are not typically encouraged to get educated about our midlife transition. If nothing is "broke," we don't necessarily feel compelled to educate ourselves, prepare ourselves, or learn about our own bodies. And if something does change to a point that it is impacting our quality of life, we've been conditioned to believe that someone "out there"—such as a doctor, health professional, pharmaceutical, or advertiser—has a magic-wand solution that will make all of our problems go away.

I mean, to a certain point, I understand this perspective. I'm not going to become an expert in diabetes, cancer, or plantar warts until I (or someone I love) is affected/diagnosed. But perimenopause and menopause don't require a diagnosis, because they are not diseases. They are merely the life phases holding up the other end of the puberty teeter-totter; phases that every woman will pass through at some point in her life.

Perimenopause and menopause, as life phases, are not revered. They are rarely discussed outside of private, hushed conversations. The word menopause is frequently misused—it is often laden with fear and certainly with negativity, surrounded by assumptions that something is "wrong" or "needs fixing." For the most part, it is misunderstood.

Since I launched MenopauseChicks.com, I've been introducing myself as a *Perimenopause Chick* or *Menopause Chick*, and I still get looks from women that say, "Oh, that doesn't apply to me." It often feels as though some women think I'm crazy for even bringing menopause up. It makes them uncomfortable. They simply do not want to talk about it, and that makes it extra challenging to ever expect our partners/spouses, friends, kids, co-workers, or even our bosses to understand the changes (or challenges) we are facing.

But here's the thing: it does apply to you—and you, and you, and you! Perimenopause and menopause are important topics, because they affect all women and represent a time of considerable growth in our lives. While not all women suffer, no one is exempt.

A friend once messaged me and said, "Shirley! Don't you dare put anything on my Facebook page. I've just started online dating, and

I don't want the world to know I have a friend in the menopause business!"

Hmmm, the menopause business. That phrase makes me giggle. See, my career has now spanned thirty years—all spent in the area of marketing, advertising, and communications. Now I almost feel like a back-stabber, as I feel compelled to call out any of my fellow advertising and copy writing colleagues who contribute to a culture that is...well...negative, and just wrong.

You see, we live in an age of communications that is predominantly based on self-doubt. And what makes matters worse is the fact that commercials—the ones my whole family watches right in the middle of *Hockey Night in Canada*—seem like they are carefully designed to scare us, and to frighten off our husbands and children too!

Advertisers work from a problem/solution formula. Think about it:

- Put on a little weight? There's an easy program for that.
- Does your bladder leak when you laugh? Someone has the solution for that.
- Trouble sleeping? They have a pill for that too.

It's not any better online. Have you tried doing your own research? "Dr. Google" is a *great* place to go at three in the morning when you can't sleep...IF you want to confirm that you are, in fact, dying!

Bookstores don't help either. I wandered around and around my local bookstore, looking for books on midlife transition. I searched through sections such as "Health" and "Women's Health" and even "Self Help," but guess where I found the books I was looking for? That's right—under a nice big sign that said **"AILMENTS & DISORDERS."**

Because of this negativity, I realized early on that my mission of simply talking about menopause was not going to be the answer. The mission had to be expanded: we needed to crack open the conversation AND re-frame menopause, if you will. We need to empower women to navigate perimenopause and menopause with as much confidence as possible. Can you imagine a future where we've redefined menopause from something that's big and ugly into a conversation women actually embrace? Where women can learn to understand the positives and the opportunities this life phase provides, can easily navigate any of its challenges, and can actually look forward to midlife? This is the future I dream of for my daughter and her friends, and their daughters.

To achieve this vision, we need to begin with trustworthy education and information. Once women are informed, proactive, and feel empowered to choose a health journey that works for them, health decisions will fall more easily into place.

I am imagining a future where women, like you, have access to awesome information, know exactly how to recruit and lead their own health care team, and—when necessary—can connect with women's health professionals to support and guide their journey.

I am imagining a time when every thirty-five-year-old woman knows what to expect, and feels prepared for perimenopause and menopause.

Definitions: Getting on the Same Page

Most books have a section at the back that provides definitions of key terms used within its pages. This isn't like most books. We are deliberately putting this section up front. While we sincerely hope you read the book from beginning to end, if there is a chance you only read (and memorize) one part of this book, please make it these next ten pages. We can't have a meaningful conversation about perimenopause and menopause unless we all begin on the same page, with a unified understanding of the terms we are talking about.

There is a quote I love by Gloria Steinam that says, "The first challenge is not to learn, but to UNlearn." This speaks to me because I've learned through thousands of conversations that it is common for women to arrive at this phase of life relatively uninformed and unprepared for what it could mean. And for many of us, before we can adequately learn about what hormone changes to expect, how to navigate perimenopause, and how to be our own best health advocates, we must first UNlearn any of the myths or misconceptions we picked up—either consciously or unconsciously—about what menopause means.

Definitions are a very important part of learning about our own health and having effective, meaningful conversations. Using the correct language is so important in helping to clear the confusing and conflicting messages around menopause.

You might think that for a life phase that every woman experiences, education for perimenopause and menopause would be common, easy to access and straight-forward. This is not the case. However, I am hopeful. As more and more women discuss their midlife health openly—and as more health professionals invest in their learning, share their expertise, and integrate their practices—perimenopause and menopause are being redefined.

For definitions, I like to refer to the life phase information as created by Dr. Jerilynn Prior at The Centre for Menstrual Cycle and Ovulation Research (CeMCOR).

As defined by CeMCOR, **Adolescence** is the time of life from the first period up to age twenty, while **premenopause** is from age twenty up to the shifts associated with perimenopause.

Perimenopause is the transition from the reproductive years to menopause. Perimenopause can begin as early as thirty-five and as late as fifty-nine, and it can last from five to fifteen years. The prefix "peri" means "around."

About ten to fifteen years before you reach menopause, your body starts giving you tiny hints that changes are coming. You may notice differences in your periods, including changes to the length, frequency, duration, or flow. If you had been keeping track, you would likely see that your length of cycle has changed from your early twenties to your mid-thirties. This occurs because maturing follicles produce less progesterone during each cycle, shortening the period of time when the uterine lining thickens in preparation for a fertilized egg.

As perimenopause begins, the number and quality of follicles diminishes to the point where not enough estrogen is produced to prompt ovulation, causing periods to become erratic—it's the mirror image of what happens when a girl first gets her period. The closer you get to the end of your reproductive years, the more changes you may notice to the duration and flow of your cycle.

Nobody told me about this—I grew up assuming menopause was like a switch, and one day your period just turned off! Isn't it fascinating that there are ads on television for erectile dysfunction and urinary incontinence, yet women in perimenopause are often surprised (and frightened) when changes occur to their period.

Although there is tremendous variation in how women progress through perimenopause—no two women are alike—it is common, as this shift happens, for women to go six to ten months between periods toward the end. There is no way to tell in advance how this may unfold for you.

Menopause is one day—it could even be a day to throw yourself a party! Natural menopause is the twelve-month anniversary of your final menstrual period. Surgical menopause is the day your ovaries are removed surgically, also known as a hysterectomy. A partial hysterectomy is the removal of the uterus only, leaving one or both ovaries in tact—so, the woman will no longer have periods, but she has not technically reached menopause yet.

Why is this important? Some women are very focused on knowing the exact countdown and definition. However, the only critical reason to know when and if you have reached menopause is if you are making birth control decisions.

In April of 2018, I attended the World Congress on Menopause, where Dr. Tim Rowe shared new information in this regard. Previously, it was pretty much a blanket statement to tell women they could no longer get pregnant if they had gone twelve months without a period—even though we knew that the twelve-month deadline was set arbitrarily and that every woman is different. Now, the guidelines for birth control indicate that if a woman is less than age fifty at the time of menopause, she should use protection for two years post-menopause. If she is fifty or older at the time of menopause, she should use protection for one year post-menopause.

The final phase to define is **post-menopause**, which is everything that comes after your anniversary party.

The reproductive life phases are often drawn in textbooks and taught in medical schools as being "black and white." This happens, and then this happens, and then this happens. The reality is that every woman's experience is unique. Many women arrive in the Menopause Chicks Private Online Community unsure about what life phase they are at. The term perimenopause was coined in 1996, so many of our mothers and grandmothers may have said "going through menopause" when they actually meant going through perimenopause and the experiences that are associated with it. You will find that health practitioners still use this terminology, and it's okay to clarify definitions with them when they do!

If you are curious, it might be helpful to draw your own timeline using these definitions. For example, I got my first period at twelve, noticed the first sign of hormonal shift (boobs hurt, brain fog, period started to change) at thirty-nine, had my last period at forty-eight (after one ten-month "pause and restart"), and reached (and celebrated!) menopause at forty-nine. Now, I am in the post-menopause phase of my life.

Many are surprised to learn just how new the term perimenopause is, and how little research actually exists on the subject. But this does help to explain how these terms can get misused—both socially and professionally. I've included some common mix-ups below.

PREmenopause Is Interchanged with PERImenopause

I find the term PREmenopause is not really used very often, except when someone is actually talking about PERImenopause. Some books also refer to this stage as the "reproductive years," but that can get confusing because you are still fertile during perimenopause. Watch for this, and seek clarification if you think the term is being used incorrectly. Most of what we talk about at MenopauseChicks.com is indeed perimenopause.

Menopause Is Interchanged for PERImenopause

This is common. I cringe when women tell me they have been told by their doctors that as long as they still have a period, it can't be menopause. While technically this is true, this is outdated thinking.

You see, many doctors were trained that women reach menopause around age fifty, and many were NOT trained in the perimenopause transition. This can mean that women get dismissed as being "too young" to be experiencing the changes that many people associate with menopause—or rather, perimenopause, as we have now learned.

Now, if you think about it, doctors should not be the ONLY resource for women looking for information on these life phases… because perimenopause and menopause are not medical conditions! They are natural life phases, just like puberty. We don't run to the doctor when a girl gets her period for the first time, unless there is something concerning. Instead, we educate and inform our girls in advance so they are prepared for the changes they face.

The same could, or should, be said about perimenopause and menopause. A helpful way to reframe our thinking and understanding is to insert the word "puberty" into a sentence where menopause or perimenopause used to be. For example, someone once said to me, "My mom didn't go through menopause." But, you would never say, "I didn't go through puberty." Therefore, a good way to clarify what that person means is to ask, "Do you mean 'she didn't suffer through menopause?'" Only 20% of women really have their worlds turned upside-down during perimenopause. Another 20% sail through with no inconveniences at all, and 60% report experiencing changes that range from mild to moderate, from inconvenient to annoying and disruptive; some temporary, others lingering.

Others might also refer to perimenopause and menopause with words such as symptoms, cure, diagnosis, and treatment. Imagine using those words when talking about puberty. It would sound weird, wouldn't it?

Whenever possible, I try to substitute the word "experiences" for "symptoms." I never get it 100% across the board, as you might notice in this book. The word "symptoms" is used when talking about disease, and menopause is not a disease. "Symptoms" is also usually synonomous with suffering, and menopause is not a synonym for suffering. Therefore, when discussing available supports for women navigating midlife health (such as treatment options and proactive health protocols), it helps to add clarity by saying "experiences associated with hormonal imbalance during perimenopause" rather than simply "menopause symptoms." It's the hormonal fluctuations and imbalances that cause symptoms, not perimenopause itself.

While defining the different phases women go through is an important first step, there are a few more definitions below that will prove helpful as you navigate your perimenopause and menopause journey.

Adrenal Glands

The adrenal glands produce important hormones—including cortisol and sex hormones—which help you respond to stress, regulate your blood pressure, control your metabolism, and more. They are located on the top of each kidney.

Tending to your adrenal health is likely where you will notice a difference between the kind of experience you might have with a family doctor versus the kind of experience you might have with a naturopathic doctor, doctor of natural medicine, or other health practitioner. Traditional medicine often does not regard the adrenals as all that important unless they completely fail or are extremely overactive, although hopefully this is changing. I had a well-respected doctor tell me there is no such thing as adrenal fatigue. In contrast, I've had numerous naturopathic doctors, and a registered nurse who is a hormone balance expert, state that taking care of our adrenals is the first priority for anyone who experiences stress (um…everyone!). Welcome to the world of confusing and conflicting information! Here's the bottom line:

- According to Dr. Sara Gottfried, adrenal fatigue is the most common hormone imbalance in women.
- Signs of adrenal issues are feeling "tired-yet-wired," sugar cravings, and abnormal weight gain.
- The best person to judge whether stress is impacting your life is YOU. Be honest. Ask questions. Get informed.

Here's my take: if you are suffering—let's say the phrase "tired-yet-wired" resonates with you—then regardless of any controversy or possible conflict with your doctor about whether or not there is such a thing as adrenal fatigue, ask if any of the following tweaks might benefit your health. They did for me.

- One step is increasing your intake of vitamins B and C. Few of us get enough B vitamins from diet alone. Consult with a health care professional about quality brands and recommended dosage. While you're at it, discuss the importance of vitamin D if you are not already taking a supplement. Most North Americans don't get adequate vitamin D from diet alone. Getting a sufficient amount of vitamin D can help with depression, improve bone strength, and prevent heart disease.
- Other suggestions include trading coffee and other sources of "fake" energy for moderate exercise, practicing mindfulness, and getting regular massages.
- I will repeat this numerous times throughout the book: do your research, get as informed as you can, and then do what's right for you.

Burnout

Why is burnout included in a list of perimenopause definitions? It's here because there's an article that's been percolating in my brain for years now. I think the title will be something like, "What if it wasn't perimenopause after all?" It may be a hard one to write after dedicating these past few years of my life to researching perimenopause and menopause, but nevertheless it's a question that I continue to ponder.

What if what I was calling signs of perimenopause were actually signs that I was burned out? I was an entrepreneur and the mother to two small children, taking care of my mother (who was living with us and exhibiting signs of dementia), and every day I was running on too much coffee and too little sleep, continuously trying to draw water from a dry well.

Do you have any idea how many other women are living the same, or similar, stress story? This is why I'm worried about women and care so strongly about being a health advocate.

I often wonder how the initial conversation with my doctor might have gone if I had said, "I'm here because I'm flat-out tired of this hamster wheel I'm on—I'm burned out," rather than, "I think I'm experiencing signs of menopause."

Burnout is a chronic stress state characterized by fatigue, headaches, disturbed sleep, pain, attention deficit, feelings of apathy and meaninglessness, and detachment from work. If this list resonates with you, please address these issues with your health care provider and take whatever proactive or reactive steps that are best for you.

Early Menopause or Surgically-Induced Menopause

This is a big topic to cover and one I don't have much personal experience with, other than witnessing my sister's early menopause. Cancer and cancer treatments is one known reason for early or premature menopause, but there are others as well.

Many women in the Menopause Chicks Private Online Community have experienced surgically-induced menopause due to a full or partial hysterectomy, and many of these women share that they were not adequately prepared by their health teams for the post-surgery hormonal changes. If you ever want to speak with someone who is knowledgeable about hormone imbalance, speak with a woman who has had a hysterectomy—many of them are experts on the subject simply because they had to figure it out for themselves, and likely had to do it in reactive mode rather than proactive.

Normal

A frequent question that arises in the Menopause Chicks Private Online Community is, "Is it normal?"

Women want to know if it is normal to experience sleep deprivation, brain fog, and moodiness; if it is normal to have heavy bleeding, rage with the people you love the most, or vertigo; if it is normal to experience anxiety, depression, vaginal dryness, and low libido.

Women like to ask if it's normal because we want to be (or need to be) validated. There is magic in knowing there are other people going through what you are experiencing. I'm here to tell you that **you are not alone**!

However, normal is not a helpful term when discussing our health. As I like to say in the Menopause Chicks Private Online Community, "Normal is a setting on your dryer." Dr. Oz has a great response to this question, where he uses an analogy for something we can all relate to: women's shoes.

You see, I wear a size 6.5, and that's considered to be within the normal range of women's shoe sizes. You might wear a size 8.5, and that's also considered normal. However, it would hurt like hell if you had to walk around all day wearing my shoes. The same applies to hormone balance, thyroid function, weight, and so on.

In short, normal for you may not be normal for me. And that is why it is upon us as bright, smart, savvy women to get as informed as we can about our own bodies, the life phases of perimenopause and menopause, and the options that are available to us, and then choose the journey that is right for us. Have I stressed that point enough?

Another way to ask the "am I normal" question is to say, "Is it common?" Often, we are simply wondering if we are the only ones going through this experience.

Placebo

A placebo is a story we tell ourselves that changes the way our brains and bodies work. Placebos are most commonly used in medical trials and treatments, where one group is given a medication that is being tested and the other is given something like a sugar pill. Sometimes, the placebo produces a 30% success rate. That's right—30% of the time, it's not the pill or the vitamin or the acupuncture or anything to do with the treatment that's improving your symptoms; it's the fact that your mind *believes* that the treatment or protocol or exercise will work.

This is why it is critically important not to judge other women for their approach to navigating their health journey. Let's say someone tells you something that can't be, or hasn't yet been, backed up by science. Perhaps they tell you "yoga helps reduce my hot flashes" or "I sleep better when I go for acupuncture or take XYZ." It doesn't matter whether those statements have been proven, because her hot flashes are reduced and she is sleeping better! Does it work, or does it work for her because she believes it will work? It simply doesn't matter.

If you've followed Menopause Chicks for a while, you will know that I am really intrigued by the placebo effect—and even the nocebo effect, which works in the opposite way. So, for example, if I tell you menopause is hell, and you believe me, there's a really good chance that menopause will be hell for you. But if I start replacing words like hot, tired, and bitchy with new words such as smart, wise, confident, and beautiful, then these word choices become my placebo for reframing perimenopause, menopause, and midlife.

Because whatever you tell yourself, you are right.

Part I

Navigating Perimenopause with Confidence and Ease

It Started with My Sister

My sister, Brenda, is ten years older than me. She is my best friend, and I have looked up to her my entire life. When it came time to learn the facts of life as I grew up, I talked to Brenda more than I talked to my mother. Sometimes, I think Mom preferred it that way; perhaps Mom understood the concept of a mokita decades before I even learned of the word!

I turned twelve in 1979, and that summer—a few months before my sister's wedding—I got my first period. I didn't tell anyone, but of course, Mom knew. She sent my sister to talk to me, and I remember the two of us counting days off on the calendar to determine if I would have my period at her wedding.

That day, I learned that Brenda didn't get her period until she was seventeen years old—the average age is twelve. You see, Brenda, is a survivor of childhood cancer, and the radiation treatments she received as a child destroyed some (but fortunately not all) of her eggs. She spent most of her teenage years either pretending she had her period, hoping her friends assumed she did, or avoiding talking about it. Menstruation is a mokita, and so is not menstruating when you are a happy, healthy teenager.

Brenda reached menopause at age thirty-six. The average age of menopause for North American Caucasian women is 51.2 years of age (the average is slightly higher for African American women, and data doesn't seem to exist for other ethnic groups); thirty-six is regarded as early or premature menopause.

It was 1992 when Brenda's periods stopped for a year, and researching health questions on the internet was not common yet. Her family doctor's response was for her to try the birth control pill. The pill brought Brenda's periods back, except instead of the two-to-three day periods she had been used to, they were now a week long with severe PMS, which she had never experienced before.

After a year on the pill, Brenda found herself discussing hormone therapy options with a gynaecologist. Perhaps the word "options" is not accurate. He said, "Your ovaries have shut down. You need to go on hormone therapy." She remembers asking why, to which he replied, "If you don't take hormone therapy, you will be putting yourself at increased risk of heart attack, cancer, and stroke, and everything will sag and dry up!" He also told Brenda she could take hormone therapy for the next twenty years and then decide how she wanted to age.

I was only twenty-six at the time, so learning about menopause was not a personal priority for me, but my sister's good health certainly was. I distinctly recall needing clarification on what her gynaecologist meant by "everything will sag and dry up." He meant that without hormone therapy, her skin and breasts would sag, and she would most likely experience vaginal dryness. As this was the first time I had even heard about this, I wasn't sure if he meant this to be less frightening or more frightening than the potential of a heart attack!

I was confident Brenda was her own best health advocate, although that's not the exact phrase I would have used back then, so when she started hormone therapy I knew it was the right choice for her. I also remember learning that our mother reached menopause at forty-nine and thinking that I had plenty of time to get informed and prepared for my own journey to menopause, and I had every intention at the time to do both.

Fast forward to 2002. The Women's Health Initiative (WHI)

study on hormone therapy (which ironically was initiated in 1991, around the time my sister and I first heard of hormone therapy) came to an abrupt halt three years early. Researchers studying the synthetic hormones Premarin and Provera determined that they were more dangerous than a placebo when given to women age sixty and over to prevent heart disease. The women in the study ranged from age fifty to seventy-one, with the average age being sixty-three. Hence, the study's results—propensity for blood clots, heart disease, stroke and breast cancer—could have been expected, as women of this age are naturally more susceptible to heart disease and breast cancer to begin with. However, the findings rocked the gynaecological world and made many physicians question the hormone therapy protocol they had been routinely prescribing to women for decades.

Without the context of the age of the participants, the study's findings made headline news. I remember even Oprah, my four o'clock goddess[1], talking about hormones. Women abruptly stopped taking their hormone therapy, and doctors and patients were left looking for a better form of relief.

The implications from the Women's Health Initiative study on women's midlife health have been vast and long-lasting. Bob Mehr, Dr. Bal Pawa and Dr. Cobi Slater explain more about this fall-out, and about viable options for women, in their chapters in Part II.

For my sister, the WHI headline news meant she needed to question her own hormone therapy protocol. "I didn't want to jeapardize my longevity," Brenda recalls. "And when I heard all the alarm bells on the news, I remember thinking—oh my god, they are talking about me!"

Now forty-six, Brenda was motivated by a conversation with her chiropractor to research all other possible options, attend workshops, and teach herself what she needed to know to make the best health decisions for her. Quitting hormone therapy cold-turkey did not seem

[1]A term of endearment borrowed from comedian Sandra Shamus; stand-up routine titled "Loss of Nouns." Search for it on YouTube. It's worth your four minutes!

like a good plan. After doing her research and advocating with her own family doctor, she decided to quit taking the synthetic hormones and transition to a plant-based estrogen and progesterone custom-made (also called "compounded") by a local pharmacy. In order to have this treatment covered by her extended medical insurance, Brenda convinced her family doctor to write the prescription.

"I felt so alone making all these decisions about my health," she says. "The information from doctors was conflicting, and I had no one to talk to about menopause or hormone therapy as none of my friends were there yet. I finally decided to trust my gut and to do what felt right."

Now fast forward to October of 2017, when the North American Menopause Society released an updated position statement declaring not only that hormone therapy remained to be the most effective treatment for vasomotor symptoms (hot flashes) and vaginal dryness, but also that it was shown to prevent bone loss and fracture[2]. To reduce the risks involved, they recommend that the treatment decisions and protocols should be individualized for each person to identify the most appropriate type, dose, formulation, route of administration, and duration of use.

It's uncanny that this chapter begins and ends on the subject of hormone therapy, as that is where many menopause conversations begin and end as well. There is so much more to learn about the perimenopause-to-menopause journey than just hormone therapy. However, for more than fifteen years, the controversy, myths, and misconceptions around hormone therapy as it relates to menopause have continued to circulate via media, marketing, and parts of the medical community. I am looking forward to a future where this subject is no longer clouded by confusing and conflicting information.

The bottom line is that for women aged sixty or younger—or who

---

[2]The 2017 hormone therapy position statement of The North American Menopause Society, The Journal of The North American Menopause Society, Volume 24, Number 7

are within ten years of menopause onset and do not have any current or high-potential risk for breast cancer, heart disease, or stroke—hormone therapy treatment has the most favourable benefit-to-risk ratio for addressing symptoms associated with hormone imbalance. This information has only been out for a year at the time this book was written, and it seems it is not yet well known or understood by women or the general medical community, except by those who have taken a special interest, special training, or who have a female-centric practice.

My sister's journey, while atypical, introduced me to these two concepts: our experiences are all unique, and the key to navigating any health question or challenge lies in learning how to be your own best health advocate.

I invite you to take Brenda's story and turn it into an invitation to navigate your own perimenopause-to-menopause-and-beyond journey with more confidence and ease. Read. Talk. Listen. Ask questions. Look in more than one place for answers. Review and revise your health plan regularly. And always, trust your instincts in order to do what is best for you and your health.

My Story, and the Story I Told Myself

On December 31, 2015, I laid in my bathtub, looked down at my body, and did something I had never done before: I thanked it.

I thanked it for allowing me to have two amazing children. I thanked it for carrying me this far on my journey. And, fairly certain that I would reach menopause in 2016, I also promised it a party.

Ten years prior, that bathtub scene had looked very different. Things were starting to change for me and I did not know what was going on in my mind or in my body, so I would retreat to the tub to try to figure out how I was going to make it through the day. Sometimes I would go to the tub to curl up in the fetal position and rock back and forth as a way to deal with the overwhelm—especially if I had just lost my cool with one of my kids for no explainable reason.

As I sat in the tub, I told myself I was a bad mother. I told myself I had to be the martyr; to take care of everyone and everything. It wasn't that I forgot to put my own name at the top of the to-do list—my own name wasn't even on the list at all! I beat myself up as I glanced at all the magazine headlines around me, most of them promising me I could lose my belly fat in just ten days. Thoughts about the potential of Alzheimer's disease danced in and out of my head. Amidst all of this turmoil, I told myself to suck it up and plunge forward. I told myself every night that tomorrow would be better, and every morning I would try to get up an hour earlier than the day before in an effort to "get it all done."

The result? I hit a wall. I suffered chronic sleep deprivation and debilitating brain fog that was affecting my ability to run my business, raise my family, and be authentically me.

Sometimes people will ask me what my first signs of perimenopause were. Looking back, I want to say it was that rogue chin hair I discovered the day of my wedding. But it is likely more accurate to say that it was sore breasts around age thirty-nine—which, in hindsight, was not that big of a deal. Of course, I didn't know at the time that fluctuating hormones were the cause, because when it comes to menopause conversations, media, marketers and the medical community have convinced us hot flashes are the first sign. This information is inaccurate and misleading and needs to be changed.

I had two healthy children, my husband had had a vasectomy, and all was good in our world. Except…my boobs hurt. Could I be pregnant? Not possible. But, I checked anyway, and the answer was no.

Over the next two to three years, other changes started happening. I experienced pronounced PMS for what seemed like the first time in my life. My periods were heavier than before I had children. I started experiencing what I now know to be perimenopausal rage, something I had never heard about at the time. I would be fine one moment, and then without warning I would come unglued and snap at the people I love the most. This was very upsetting. Then came the brain fog, which was frustrating. I could make a list, but all I could do was stare at it; I couldn't seem to accomplish what I used to in a day. I was having trouble remembering things—simple things like people's names, cupcake day at the kids' school, and my suitcase at the airport. I lacked focus, which was really scary as a self-employed entrepreneur. I also had a low libido, but we are a busy family so it felt legitimate and understandable that I didn't seem to have the time or energy I once had. Besides, I was awake every day at 3:00 a.m.!

Now, I'm not the kind of person who goes to the doctor for every little thing; in fact, I don't really go to the doctor much at all. But after noticing these changes for a couple of years, I decided to mention that I was possibly experiencing the first signs of menopause (I wasn't aware of the term perimenopause yet) to my doctor...at the end of my Pap smear appointment. While I'm not a huge fan of medical procedures, I really don't mind this test at all; it's preventative and necessary.

My doctor was lovely, but besides helping to deliver my two healthy babies, we really haven't talked that much over the years. However, I still went in with a preconceived idea that if there ever was something concerning to me that I wanted to discuss, the conversation would be directional, informative, validating, and above all, supportive.

So, there I was, lying on her examining table post-Pap, donning a lovely, blue, paper-thin gown the size of a Post-it note. My doctor says, "Go ahead and sit up. Is there anything else?"

I was crunched forward, trying to strategically position the Post-it. I felt vulnerable and unprepared—and a little bit like a teenage girl—as I conjured up the courage to say the word "menopause" for the first time. I stammered out, "Well, actually I wanted to ask you...errr...well, I'm just wondering...you see, I think I might be experiencing the first signs of menopause."

It felt strange to say the word. I was embarrassed at how little I knew. I was in denial that I might be "that old." I was sad to think my reproductive years were coming to an end. And I was scared. I really, *really* wanted to rule out the idea that I might be experiencing early-onset dementia.

She looked at me, and then looked at the birthdate on my chart. "Oh, you're forty-one," she quipped. "You're too young for menopause."

You might think that would make me feel better. It did not. At first I thought, *Whew, what a relief,* but that was quickly followed by, *Wait a second—if it's not that, what is it?*

I know my doctor went on to say something about birth control pills, sleeping pills, and anti-depressants, but I couldn't hear her because my internal voice was screaming, *SHIRLEY, SUCK IT UP! THIS IS ALL IN YOUR HEAD!*

If you are reading this and thinking "damn doctor" or anything of that nature, I beg you to stop. Yes, I was disappointed at how that particular conversation left me with more questions than answers, but it is not my doctor's fault. Do not fire your doctor simply because your initial conversation about perimenopause or menopause doesn't meet your expectations! Also, do not assume that a female doctor will meet your needs better than a male one—this is a common misconception, and you must remember that both were educated beside each other in medical school. You need your family physician. However, you may need to change how you form your expectations and approach your conversations about your midlife or hormonal health. Knowing what options your doctor (or other midlife health professional) has in his or her toolkit is an important first step. That is why we have included thirteen chapters in part II of this book to help you build the midlife health team that is right for you.

I made a decision after that doctor's visit: my midlife journey was my responsibility. Yes, I did feel confused, and even embarrassed, after that particular conversation. But the more I thought about it, the more I wondered if I was the only woman in the world feeling this way.

Life remained busy, and my experiences of perimenopause ebbed and flowed throughout my early forties. By the age of forty-six, I embarked on some research. I became obsessed with the lack of quality information and online conversations for women to prepare themselves for perimenopause and menopause—at least in the same way we all prepare our children for puberty! And I was driven to fill the gap for women trying to navigate this journey as I was. I wanted to crack open the conversation so women would feel more informed and less alone.

And that was the beginning of MenopauseChicks.com

Your story will be different from mine. You may be wondering the same things I did, or you may have questions of your own. Being your own health advocate means finding the answers to those questions and being willing to talk about what you are experiencing.

Hormones: Clearing up Their Bad Reputation

Prior to starting MenopauseChicks.com, I admit that the word "hormones" felt like a swear word; whenever it landed on my ears, it came with a negative connotation.

An eye-rolling teenager often prompts statements like "oh, she's hormonal" or "the hormones are raging!" I heard people talking about "hormone imbalances" and how their "hormones are out of whack." Even two of my favourite experts wrote books called *The Hormone Cure* and *The Hormone Diet*—both with titles (not content) that paint hormones in a less-than-desirable light.

It's time to flip the conversation and talk about hormones in a positive context! Hormones are our friends; they deserve our attention and love, because they have important jobs to do.

Here is a brief hormone primer courtesy of Dr. Sara Gottfried, author of *The Hormone Cure*.

Androgens are the class of hormones that stimulate male characteristics by binding to androgen receptors on cells. Even though women have far lower levels of androgens than men, we are exquisitely sensitive to androgen levels and need to maintain the proper amount for optimal health. Having an improper amount of androgens in your system affects your vitality, confidence, and lean body mass. Ovarian overproduction of androgens is a condition in which the ovaries make too much testosterone and is linked to polycystic ovarian syndrome.

This condition can lead to a woman developing male characteristics such as rogue hairs, acne, or hair loss.

Cortisol is produced by the adrenal glands. It plays a role in your bones, circulatory system, immune system, nervous system, stress responses, and the metabolism of fats, carbohydrates, and proteins. While each hormone has a job, Dr. Gottfried refers to estrogen, thyroid, and cortisol as the top three most essential hormones, with cortisol being number one. High cortisol causes you to feel tired-but-wired and prompts your body to store fuel as fat in places it can be used easily, such as at your waist. Low cortisol makes you feel exhausted and drained, like a car trying to run on an empty gas tank.

DHEA is an abbreviation for dehydroepiandrosterone. It affects your mood and sex drive, can convert into testosterone when needed, and is a member of the androgen family. Too much DHEA has been associated with depression and acne.

Estrogen refers to a family of hormones (estradiol, estriol, and estrone) that are produced primarily in the ovaries (before menopause) to promote female characteristics such as breast growth and menstruation. Estrogen affects your libido, mood, joints, and mental state. High estrogen makes you more likely to develop breast tenderness, cysts, fibroids, endometriosis, and breast cancer. Low estrogen causes your mood and libido to tank and makes your vagina less moist, your joints less flexible, and your mental state less focused and alive.

Progesterone is released by your ovaries, and its role is to stimulate the uterus to prepare for pregnancy. A low amount of progesterone can cause anxiety, night sweats, sleeplessness, and irregular cycles.

Testosterone is often thought of as a male hormone; however, it is vital for women as well. Testosterone is the hormone responsible for vitality and self-confidence, but producing too much testosterone is the main reason for female infertility. Testosterone is linked to your sex drive, and too little testosterone results in low libido in both women and men.

Leptin regulates hunger and metabolism and helps our body adjust how we burn fat.

Insulin drives glucose into our cells to be used as fuel and deposits fat. Chronically high insulin increases estrogen and our cells' resistance to insulin.

Thyroid is often thought of as the gland responsible for metabolism, energy, weight, and mood, but it also refers to the hormones produced by this gland. When it is healthy, your thyroid produces hormones (TSH, T4, T3, T2, T1, and reserve T3) in the correct amounts to make you feel energetic, think clearly, and be upbeat. Low thyroid hormone (also known as hypothyroid) is characterized by feelings of sluggishness and poor memory. Many women misinterpret these feelings as simply signs of getting older, but it's not just aging! Instead of just accepting them, have your thyroid checked. Fifteen to twenty percent of women with depression are low in thyroid hormone. Hyperthyroid (also known as an overactive thyroid or too much thyroid hormone) is less common, affecting approximately 2% of women, and causes experiences such as heart palpitations, shortness of breath, and weight loss.

Women have a 20% chance of developing a thyroid issue—either too high or too low—at some point in their lives. That statistic alone is too important to ignore, so please investigate if this situation applies to you!

Vitamin D is considered both a hormone and a vitamin. It is responsible for bone strength and for fighting off depression and heart disease. It can be made by mammals when they are exposed to the sun; the challenge is that many North Americans do not get enough sun exposure, so we are vitamin D deficient. As a result, taking a vitamin D supplement is strongly recommended for everyone.

In summary, cortisol gives us focus while thyroid keeps us energized, comfortably warm, and at a manageable weight. Estrogen has over 300 jobs in a woman's body including regulating menstruation and keeping us juicy, from our joints to our vaginas. Progesterone regulates the uterine lining, emotions, and sleep. Testosterone is responsible for vitality and self-confidence. Leptin controls our hunger. Insulin regulates how we use fuel from food. Vitamin D has a number of roles, including promoting bone strength and fighting depression and heart disease.

While I do imagine a day when every woman is armed with hormone education before her thirty-fifth birthday, I am finding that women currently learn about hormones as they begin to fluctuate—most often in perimenopause. I know that was true for me.

When I started perimenopause, I was feeling burned out, had difficulty concentrating, felt anxious and depressed for the first time in my life, and was chronically sleep-deprived. However, I didn't even know the names of my hormones, much less how they might relate to what I was going through.

When I sat down with my naturopath, Dr. van Drimmelen (you can read her chapter starting on 207), near the end of 2015, my biggest concerns were anxiety, depression, and difficulty concentrating. She pulled out a rating chart and asked me to assign a number to each experience, where zero meant not at all and five meant extreme. Using my ratings, she was able to formulate the best plan of action (including testing, a vitamin and supplement regimen, and bioidentical hormone therapy). For me, I really appreciated learning which hormone was responsible for which experience.

Here is what I learned from Dr. van Drimmelen's rating chart. I hope it is helpful to you—as an educational tool, a checklist, a benchmark to help you identify where you are on your own journey, or something you can use in conversation with your health care professional. Remember—health care professionals are scientists and they appreciate visual evidence to support your story. Tracking your experiences will go a long way in helping your doctor help you! You might use a checklist or a rating scale—anything that will help you communicate your experiences better.

Fluctuations in **progesterone** may contribute to:

- Difficulty concentrating
- Moodiness/emotional swings
- Depressed or unhappy feelings
- Anxious
- Headaches
- Difficulty sleeping
- Painful or swollen breasts
- Weight gain/bloating
- PMS
- Heavy bleeding

Fluctuations in **estrogen** may contribute to:

- Night sweats
- Difficulty remembering things
- Hot flashes
- Vaginal dryness
- Dry hair/skin
- Incontinence
- Frequent urinary tract infections
- Low libido
- Painful intercourse

Fluctuations in **testosterone** may contribute to:

- Loss of libido
- Lack of desire to be intimate
- Loss of motivation
- Flat mood
- Diminished well-being
- Blunted emotion

Fluctuations in **thyroid** hormone may contribute to:

- Fatigue/exhaustion
- Cold hands and feet/low body temperature
- Weight gain or inability to lose weight

- Constipation
- Depressed or unhappy feelings
- Dry skin/nails/hair or hair loss
- Poor concentration
- Muscle aches and pains
- Puffy eyes/face
- Low libido

Fluctuations in **cortisol** may contribute to:

- Feeling stressed
- Insomnia
- Tired-yet-wired
- Irritability
- Lightheaded if meal is missed
- Frequent colds/flu
- Anxious
- Depressed/unhappy
- Weight gain (waist)
- Fatigue/exhaustion
- Food cravings
- Aches and pains
- Chronic health problems such as diabetes or pre diabetes

I have spoken with a number of women who are frustrated because their physicians don't see the value in testing hormone levels. This is a common story. It is important to know that testing hormone levels is only one tool a health professional has to determine the best protocol for you and your particular situation. However, if you are interested in hormone testing and experiencing resistance from your doctor, there are some approaches you can try to get him or her to reconsider. In *The Hormone Cure*, Dr. Sara Gottfried offers these suggestions to use in your conversation:

- "I just read a book about hormone balance and learned a lot.

Because I'm experiencing [insert yours], I'm wondering if you'd be willing to order a blood test for me?"

- If your doctor declines certain testing, be polite yet assertive. "I've read there's a link between [fill in the blank with your experience] and [fill in the blank with hormone]. I'd really like to pursue testing to get to the bottom of this." Or, "Can you please explain why it's not worthwhile to test?"
- If your doctor continues to refuse, you might ask if he or she can refer you to someone who'd be willing to order the tests.

Estrogen Dominance

Traditionally, menopause has been associated with estrogen deficiency. Women were led to believe that at the first sign of symptoms, they should run out and get an estrogen replacement. While estrogen does fluctuate in perimenopause, it doesn't fall significantly until after your final period. Far more women actually suffer from what is known as estrogen dominance during their perimenopause-to-menopause transition. Estrogen dominance is very common in women and begins as early as age thiry-five.

Estrogen dominance is when you have too much estrogen relative to progesterone. When a woman's menstrual cycle is normal, estrogen is the dominant hormone for the first two weeks leading up to ovulation, then is balanced by progesterone during the last two weeks. As a woman enters perimenopause and begins to experience anovulatory cycles (that is, cycles where no egg is released), estrogen can often go unopposed, causing symptoms to appear.

How might you know if you are estrogen dominant? According to Dr. Christiane Northrup, author of *The Wisdom of Menopause*, any of the following symptoms could indicate estrogen dominance:

- Decreased sex drive
- Irregular menstrual periods

- Bloating
- Breast swelling and tenderness
- Fibrocystic breasts
- Headaches
- Mood swings (most often irritability and depression)
- Weight gain (particularly around the abdomen and hips)
- Cold hands and feet (also a symptom of thyroid dysfunction)
- Hair loss
- Sluggish metabolism
- Foggy thinking, memory loss
- Fatigue
- Trouble sleeping
- PMS

By the way, all of these symptoms can also be brought on by excessive stress (which leads to adrenal exhaustion), which is why it is always important to consult a health care professional to get a better picture of your overall health.

When it comes to decreasing estrogen dominance, Dr. Northrup recommends several potential steps:

- **Improve your diet:** You can increase the amount of nutrients in your diet by taking a high-potency multivitamin/mineral combination. You can also start following a hormone-balancing diet, which includes eating lots of fresh fruits and vegetables, adequate protein, and moderate amounts of healthy fat. Getting enough fibre in your diet is also important as estrogen is excreted by the bowels, and if stool remains in the bowels due to constipation then estrogen can be reabsorbed into your system. Losing excess body fat and getting regular exercise, especially strength training, will also be beneficial.
- **Consider natural, bioidentical progesterone:** Progesterone cream is available over-the-counter in the United States

and by prescription in Canada. Many symptoms of estrogen dominance can be relieved with natural, bioidentical progesterone, available in a 2% cream (one-quarter teaspoon contains about twenty milligrams of progesterone). Use one-quarter to one-half teaspoon of 2% progesterone cream on your skin (face, breasts, abdomen, and hands) daily for two to three weeks prior to onset of period. If your periods are irregular, use 2% progesterone daily, or from the full moon to the dark of the moon.

- Talk with your health care provider about ways to **detoxify your liver:** Traditional Chinese Medicine explains that symptoms of estrogen dominance are caused by blocked liver and kidney chi. The liver acts as a filter, helping us screen out the harmful effects of toxins from our environment and the products we put in our bodies. When the liver has to work hard to eliminate toxins such as alcohol, drugs, caffeine, or environmental agents, the liver's capacity to cleanse the blood of estrogen is compromised.
- **Decrease stress:** Paying close attention to how to manage stress will also be beneficial. Practice saying no to excessive demands on your time. Remember, perimenopause is an opportunity to reinvent yourself. This means investing time and energy in yourself, not everyone else.

Determining If Hormone Therapy Is Right for You

First of all, hear this: hormone therapy is not the one and only solution. Dr. Christiane Northrup, explains it is an individual choice. Here are Dr. Northrup's recommended list of things to consider.

- How much do you need relief from current discomfort, particularly hot flashes and lack of sleep?

- Are you suffering from urinary incontinence?
- How is your heart health; what are your risk factors for cardiovascular disease?
- Are you at an increased risk for osteoporosis?
- Are you at an increased risk for Alzheimer's?
- Are you at an increased risk for breast, uterine, ovarian, or bowel cancer?
- Did you reach menopause prematurely (before forty) or artificially and abruptly (due to surgery, illness, chemotherapy, or radiation)?

Your answers to these questions will help you figure out whether hormone therapy will be a safe and effective course of action for you.

On top of these considerations, consider creating a lifestyle protocol before turning to hormone therapy. Hormone imbalances can be tweaked by paying attention to how we eat, move, and sleep. If that alone doesn't do the trick, consider working with a professional who can recommend vitamins and supplements to support your midlife transition. If that doesn't work, *then* have a conversation about the potential of hormone therapy and how that might address your current concerns. Be sure to discuss bioidentical versus synthetic hormones, dosage recommendations, possible side effects, how your therapy will be measured and monitored, and what the recommended exit strategy will be.

Hormones are what make our bodies work. By learning about what they do, and about the signs of hormone imbalances, we can take further control of our own health journey.

Cracking Open the Conversation

Since April 2016, we've cracked open over 240,000 conversations in the Menopause Chicks Private Online Community. The most common topics from our website and private community are:

1. Adrenal health
2. Bleeding
3. Brain fog
4. Hot flashes and night sweats
5. Navigating perimenopause and marriage at the same time

These, along with other popular topics—such as sexual health, pelvic health, mental and emotional health, and sleep—are discussed in Part II by our women's health professionals. For now, I will give you an overview of these five topics through excerpts from the most popular posts in our community.

1. Adrenal Health

From an interview with Cathy McCann, McCann Nutrition

Many women are unaware of the importance of adrenal health, and particularly of how it can impact their journey through perimenopause.

What is adrenal fatigue?

Our adrenal glands are designed to protect us from physical harm–for example, from a saber-toothed tiger. They help send all available energy to our muscles to fight off the danger. This means they are very important in managing our stress response system in the short-term, but they can be very damaging if they are tapped for extended periods of time. The challenge is that most of us are NOT fighting off real tigers, although it often feels that way! Instead, many of us are juggling work and family—taking care of older and younger family members, attempting to please crabby bosses, fighting traffic, fighting financial stress, and fighting with our spouses. Our bodies can't tell the difference between real physical stress and perceived stress, so it responds to modern-day stressors in the same way it would respond to the pouncing tiger.

Women tend to spend much of the first half of their lives nourishing and giving to others. In their second half, women need to learn how to nourish, heal, and thrive in their own lives.

How do our adrenals affect our perimenopause-to-menopause journey?

Healthy adrenal glands release small amounts of estrogen and progesterone; at menopause, they are designed to take over for our ovaries and ease our way through the transition. But if our adrenals are worn out...BAM! There's a good chance the perimenopause journey may include experiences such as insomnia, reduced sex drive, and that tired-yet-wired feeling, because our adrenals are tapped out.

Why does it seem like no one is talking about this?

There seems to be a growing number of conversations about perimenopause and menopause, and adrenal health is becoming a more popular topic (although there is still a long way to go). What seems to be missing from the conversation is the realization and understanding of how interconnected and dependent one is on the other. We have made the connection between adrenals and stress management. Now, by bringing awareness of the connection between adrenals and hormone health, we are finally understanding that adrenal health is one of the main ingredients—if not THE main ingredient—to a smooth perimenopause journey!

What can women do to optimize adrenal health?

An important first step is to **manage your stress**. It sounds so cliche, but this is really, really important. Put your own name at the top of your to-do list and consider meditation, yoga, exercise, human connection (hugging, sex, time with friends), time in nature, whatever brings you joy.

You also need to **focus on nutrition**. Eat more whole foods and less processed foods. Pay attention to your vitamin and mineral needs. Talk with a professional about vitamin B and C and magnesium. You may also discuss options for some herbs that support your adrenals, such as ashwaganda—often prescribed for stress and fatigue and proven to increase energy and improve longevity.

2. Changes to Bleeding

As progesterone begins to fluctuate, women in perimenopause often experience changes to their monthly periods—they may get heavier or lighter, longer or shorter, less frequent or more frequent. This is a common experience, but it isn't yet common knowledge.

We have a tendency to associate menopause with hot flashes. However, while hot flashes and night sweats can be disruptive to a woman's quality of life, there are many other changes that don't get as much airtime.

According to the International Menopause Society, abnormal bleeding accounts for 70% of all gynaecological visits. Women might be less worried about these changes if they knew what to expect; that being said, consulting your health care practitioner for bleeding that's different in frequency, regularity, duration, or amount is always a good idea, for no other reason than to rule out more serious concerns such as fibroids or cancer. You should always consult a doctor for:

- bleeding that is so heavy it requires a new pad every hour
- bleeding that lasts more than two weeks
- any bleeding after menopause (twelve months after your final period)

The Centre for Menstrual Cycle and Ovulation Research advises women with heavy flow to keep track of their experience (to discuss with their doctor if necessary), to take 200 mg of ibuprofen every four to six hours (which decreases flow by 25-30%), to treat blood loss with extra fluid and salt, and to increase your intake of iron with iron-rich foods or a supplement (consult your physician or pharmacist for guidance).

3. Brain Fog

Brain fog is a common complaint of women in perimenopause, and I can certainly relate. When I first noticed brain fog, I was a self-employed thirty-nine-year-old mother of two young children. I could not focus. I would write lists—and re-write lists—in fear of forgetting something, but all I could do was stare at the words in my notebook for hours. It was as if my brain had forgotten how to propel those words into action.

On many occasions, I would give up and go to bed, vowing to

get up early tomorrow and "make it happen." Only, I quickly realized that the brain fog followed me from day to day to day, often bringing with it sleep deprivation, forgetfulness, and moodiness like I had never experienced before. I didn't know how to describe what I was experiencing, or what to call it.

My livelihood depends on my ability to function at a high level, to think clearly, and to formulate articulate thoughts, and it was being impacted by this fog. This wasn't the procrastination I experienced in university, when I chose going out with friends over writing a paper. This was me—for the first time in my life—feeling off the rails. I convinced myself that I must be the only one going through this. I put on a brave face to the rest of the world and acted as if I was okay, but inside I felt like I was losing my ability to be the high-functioning, always-on woman I knew and still wanted to be.

My nurse and hormone expert, Debbie Brown, introduced me to the benefits of magnesium and vitamins B, C, and D. She encouraged me to take better care of myself, and I found that improvements to my sleep—and, more importantly, to how I felt when I was awake—really helped with putting the brain fog at bay.

The problem is, I'm not always a super compliant patient. Fast-forward to six years later and brain fog reared its ugly head again, this time accompanied by depression and a growing lack of self-trust from my inability to concentrate. I was forgetting important tasks and missing flights. I revisited Debbie's supplement recommendations and started on my journey to learn which hormones are responsible for what. I learned that difficulty with concentration can be the product of fluctuating progesterone in perimenopause, and difficulty remembering things can be related to fluctuating estrogen. Poor concentration can also be related to an imbalance in thyroid hormone.

Two-thirds of women cite brain fog as being one of the most frustrating perimenopause symptoms. Look at any list of described experiences for perimenopause and you'll find terms such as fuzzy thinking, tired-yet-wired, forgetfulness, and decreased problem-solving ability. Women complain about "cotton head," the inability to concentrate, and forgetting people's names and common nouns.

There are two theories about where brain fog comes from:

- **Hormonal changes:** The ovaries no longer produce the same consistent levels of estrogen and progesterone that they used to, and the brain is less responsive to the hormones your ovaries do still produce.
- **Other perimenopausal symptoms:** Mood swings, anxiety/depression, chronic overwhelm, and poor sleep can all lead to mental fuzziness.

So, what can be done about brain fog? First, it is important to review any and all changes in your health with your health care provider, if for no other reason than to rule out other concerns. Track your symptoms leading up to your appointment so your physician has a clear picture of what is normal versus abnormal for you.

Next, explore strategies that fit your own personal health care journey. This could mean talking with a naturopath about hormone level testing and supplementation recommendations. It might mean seeking out the advice of an acupuncturist; a number of studies show that acupuncture can increase blood flow and brain function and relieve many of the symptoms associated with perimenopause.

Review your lifestyle habits, such as diet, nutrition, sleep, and exercise. Are there tweaks to be made? Chances are you already know the answers to some of the key questions that could improve—or even eliminate—your brain fog.

1. How is your diet? Are you getting enough leafy greens and omega-3-rich foods?
2. What are you drinking? Too much caffeine? Too much alcohol? Not enough water? Adequate hydration is vital for the brain to function properly.

3. When was the last time you broke a sweat? Exercise automatically boosts the "feel good" brain chemicals like serotonin and helps to regulate both mood and cognitive function.
4. Are there any new strategies you'd be willing to introduce, such as yoga or meditation?
5. How much sleep are you getting?

Finally, try to have perspective; take time to breathe, to forgive yourself, and to know that you are likely not in the early stages of dementia. Even the most extreme moments of brain fog are probably temporary.

4. Hot Flashes and Night Sweats

The most common and most talked about experience of perimenopause, menopause, and beyond are hot flashes.

Did you know the actual term is "hot FLUSH"?

We took the question of what to do about hot flashes to Dr. Jerilynn Prior, MD, Professor of Endocrinology at the University of British Columbia and founder of the Centre for Menstrual Cycle and Ovulation Research. In her reply below, she correctly uses "flush" instead of "flash." It is just another one of those quirky things about navigating this topic and figuring out all the confusing and conflicting info.

> For night sweats and hot flushes, what I recommend as the most natural—and therefore least harmful—therapy is **anything that decreases your feeling of stress**. There is good evidence to support what is called "paced breathing," which is a kind of meditation or relaxation therapy that uses slow, deep, controlled breathing. Sit in a quiet place with your body relaxed and your eyes closed, and first become aware of your breathing.

Then slowly take a deep breath in, and equally slowly let it out. You might count as you breathe in, perhaps up to ten. Let your breath out without any effort, say to a count of five or six. Focus on your breath and nothing else.

Alternate methods of relaxation are to sit in the same quiet place and relaxed manner, and to visualize yourself in the most calm, secure, and lovely place you can imagine. If you practice, you will be able to smell the air, feel the breeze on your face, and see the whole full-colour environment. For these relaxation and breathing methods to be effective, you will need to do them for ten to twenty minutes twice a day. One good time to do this is just before going to sleep. If you practice, you will be able to capture the same calm in the middle of a busy day.

In addition to these methods of decreasing your stress responses, it's a good idea to see if there are any ways you can lighten your load or deal with the things that are bothering you. If I am under great stress, my night sweats return no matter how hard I try to relax.

The second option is an herbal product called **black cohosh** which is marketed as "Remifemin." The four papers that have tested this for treating hot flushes/night sweats used different doses, but it looks like four milligrams twice a day is the effective dose, although you should always read the package label. It has one disadvantage—it has some estrogen-like activity and therefore may not be safe for long-term use (in other words, for more than six months). For example, two of the two studies that tested the effect of black cohosh on the vagina found it acted like estrogen and therefore may make vaginal dryness better. However, that means there are also risks for breast tenderness, breast lumps, and possibly breast cancer as well as for vaginal bleeding or unwanted periods.

Vitamin E (400 IU once or twice a day) has been tested for hot flushes in only one recent trial and was statistically stronger than a placebo. However, there may be other reasons to take vitamin E, and it is also likely to be safe. So, you could begin with 400 IU a day while working on your breathing!

I believe that night sweats that persistently waken you from sleep need to be treated; otherwise, there are adverse effects on mood, muscle and joint symptoms, and potentially other problems such as increased bone loss. If you try these natural therapies and they are not sufficient to prevent night sweats, then I would recommend **progesterone.** There is one trial showing that progesterone cream, when used in a dose of twenty milligrams per day, improves hot flushes in women who have reached menopause. Whether this dose is helpful in perimenopause is not known. Progesterone cream is only available via a doctor's prescription in Canada, but is available over the counter in the United States.

My preference would be **oral micronized progesterone (Prometrium)**, which is bioidentical to your ovary's own progesterone. It is available in 100-milligram round capsules that look like beige salmon eggs. They are made with peanut oil to increase absorption, and therefore should be avoided by those allergic to peanuts or other nuts. Progesterone should be taken just before going to bed because the oral medication has an excellent side effect of causing drowsiness. It may also cause some dizziness for the first two to three hours after first taking it. This is not a serious side effect and shouldn't worry you—just lie down and go peacefully to sleep.

The Prometrium dose that I know to be effective for night sweats in perimenopause is 300 milligrams taken daily at bedtime. It does not cause vaginal bleeding, breast tenderness, depression, weight gain, migraines, or acne. The drug books that indicate that these are progesterone side effects are, for medical-legal reasons, referring to everything that has been noted with estrogen and male-hormone derived progestins that are in birth control pills.

If you prefer to use a natural progesterone cream, you should ask for a prescription from your doctor for a dose of 100 milligrams twice a day. Ask around for a compounding pharmacy that can make this for you. Be sure that they supply it with a measuring device and tell you how many milligrams there are in one unit of measure. The dose can safely be increased if needed.

For more information, please visit Dr. Prior's website at The Centre for Menstrual Cycle and Ovulation Research (CeMCOR.ubc.ca). CeMCOR is not-for-profit and relies on donations to carry out critical research on women's health.

5. Perimenopause, Menopause, and Marriage

According to Statistics Canada, divorce among those fifty-five and over has been steadily growing, and is expected to increase as our population continues to age. Sixty-six percent of these divorces are initiated by women who are in their forties, fifties, and sixties. (AARP/CARP)

Now, I'm not saying there is a direct correlation between menopause and divorce, because there are many interpersonal factors and nuances that make up a relationship. We do know, however, that any time significant change is happening for one person—be it career, family, emotional, or physical—there is a direct impact on their partner.

Menopause and perimenopause are no exception.

This does not mean that perimenopause and menopause are

universally bad for your marriage. These are life phases that women can successfully navigate with loving support from their family, friends, health care providers, and community. Marriage and/or significant partnerships often provide the pinnacle of that support.

Here are a few recommendations to help you help your husbands/partners/loved ones navigate the menopausal years with you.

Sort out fact from fiction

Menopause means old. Menopause makes you crazy or sick. Menopause can be reversed. These are all fiction! The truth is that hormone levels begin to change as early as thirty-five, and perimenopause can last up to fifteen years. The average age of menopause is fifty-one. Eighty percent of women experience symptoms during perimenopause, ranging from mild to severe. Some women seek treatments to manage their symptoms, while others manage them with a healthy diet, sleep, and physical activity. It's helpful to begin your conversations about menopause with the basic facts so there are no preconceived notions getting in the way of finding the journey that's best for you.

Know what you don't know

There is no need to feel ashamed or stupid; it's not as if they teach this subject at school! Menopause is one of life's most confusing and misunderstood transitions—for men, women, and even some health care professionals. It's possible that you are learning about this life phase at the exact same time as your partner. The important thing is for both of you to remain curious, ask questions, seek clarification, and keep the lines of communication open. Avoidance and denial will only get in the way.

Find the right language

As you are finding your way through the midlife maze, you may be seeking solutions for your experiences (or "symptoms") or their root causes. This, along with various messages from the media, could leave your partner with the wrong impression—that menopause is a disease, an ailment, something that requires fixing or a cure. This couldn't be further from the truth. When you use the right language and frame your experience in the right context, it will be easier for your loved ones to do the same when they are talking to other friends, family members, or even their buddies.

Abracadabra phrases

You probably have a few "magic phrases" that already work in your relationship. For example, whenever my hubby refrains from trying to fix whatever I'm complaining about and gives me a genuine "I understand," I immediately calm down. Ask your partner/husband to dust off the phrases he/she knows work for you, and to have them at the ready.

No joking matter

There's so much room for a great sense of humour during our midlife years. While it is sometimes validating to joke around with girlfriends about our forgetfulness, facial hair, or inability to jump on a trampoline like we used to, it can be humiliating to be the punch line of someone else's joke. One way to address this is to chat about your own personal preferences—lovingly and privately—before it happens.

You might want to kill him/her at some point

It might not be his/her fault—or, maybe it is! There's potential for a wide range of symptoms to wreak havoc in your life. These include brain fog, PMS, mood swings, depression, irritability, rage, hot flashes and night sweats, weight gain, sleep deprivation, and sudden bouts of not being able to remember where you parked the car. If you find yourself in a moment (or week) of feeling off-kilter and lashing out at the people who love you the most, be sure to name what is happening rather than hiding it. Helpful phrases can include:

- "I'm irritable because I'm not sleeping properly."
- "Please be kind—I can't think straight today and it's really overwhelming."
- "I'm not feeling like myself today."

Vaginal dryness is not the same as lack of interest

Help your partner understand that lower libido and vaginal dryness are common experiences of perimenopause and menopause, not a sign that you don't love him anymore. When our vehicles get low on oil, we don't desert them; we tend to them and give them what they need to run optimally. The same tender loving care is required for our bodies too. It's important he knows you are still very interested in him, and in lovemaking. Hormonal or non-hormonal treatments are easy to access via your doctor and/or pharmacy. A little lubrication, plus a large dose of "vitamin O" (orgasms), is proven to lower stress, lower cortisol, reduce anxiety, and help women sleep better and feel more connected.

No matter what you are experiencing in your perimenopause-to-menopause-and-beyond journey, there are lots of supports available to you. Do your research and find the options that work best for you!

Myths, Misconceptions, and Media Innuendo

Marie Osmond steps onto a stage in a television commercial for incontinence pads and proclaims all women leak a little when they laugh. A google search for menopause or perimenopause only returns images of gray-haired women holding fans. Media writers lump menopause stories in with chronic conditions by using words such as ailments, disorders, disease, condition, diagnose, cure, and treatment.

We've all been subjected to the myths, misconceptions, and media innuendo that accompanies menopause. In North American society in particular, we've adopted these negative connotations that are passed onto us, both culturally and generationally. As a result, somewhere along the line we learned that menopause is something that must be either feared or fixed.

When I speak with someone about menopause, typically the first words they come up with have to do with "struggling." Rarely does someone respond with positive words like smart, confident, or free. Yet neither perimenopause or menopause are synonyms for suffering; they are life phases on a woman's reproductive road map, just like puberty. I believe that this is because we are so used to seeing the stereotypical image of the stressed-out lady who can't sleep or doesn't want to have sex with her husband that many of us just assume that's an accurate representation of menopause. And it's one we want to run away from rather than embrace. But when I call myself a *Menopause Chick*, it helps to strip away the (negative) power; then, I can choose to reframe menopause from something that is solely negative into a milestone worth celebrating!

In my 2016 TEDx Talk, I told the story of finding my favourite magazine in an airport with the headline "Hooray for Hormones!" I was so excited that there was finally a publication putting a positive spin on hormone health, only to open up the pages to images telling women they can expect to get fat, hot, lose their memories, and lose control of their bladders in their thirties, forties, and fifties. I looked at the magazine photos and thought, *Are these the new profile pictures for menopause?* That's when I realized it's not menopause that fascinates me; it's what women are willing to put up with.

There's some good news happening, and I can feel that change is imminent. But it will take all of us speaking up—with our voices and our wallets—to turn the big ol' dinosaur around. Here are a few movements I'm excited to watch and support:

- In September 2017, Allure magazine banned the term "anti-aging," acknowledging that growing older is something that should be embraced and appreciated rather than resisted.
- #SeeHer (spearheaded by the Association of National Advertisers) is a movement that honours the fact that over 60% of female consumers believe women are commonly depicted using negative stereotypes in ads (A & E Networks). Their mission is to increase the accurate portrayals of women and girls in US advertising and media 20% by the year 2020. I am looking forward to more accurate portrayals for many reasons, including the fact that this is a growing demographic. In 2005, there were 477 million post-menopausal women in the world. By 2025, that number will jump to 1.1 billion.
- McCann Advertising in Canada and Super Human in the UK—both ad agencies—are working to ensure brands can better connect with women in midlife by eradicating outdated messaging and media innuendo around ageism. Both agencies

have conducted extensive research studies and discovered women in midlife are keenly interested in health, education and adventure. We no longer want the manufacturers we buy from or the media programming we subscribe to to view menopause as an obstacle. Instead, women in midlife want menopause elevated as an important life stage worthy of acceptance, acknowledgement, honour, and celebration.

* McCann is the author of a series of studies called The Truth About Canadian Women. An excerpt from their report on "The Truth About Canadian Women Over 50: The Untapped Opportunity" can be viewed at TruthAboutCanadianWomen.ca.
* Super Human conducted a UK-wide survey in 2018 designed to show advertisers how attitudes toward menopause are changing. You can learn more at WeAreSuperHuman.co.uk.

Changing how the media portrays menopause is important if we want to create a future where women no longer feel alone in their experiences, where they feel more comfortable talking about perimenopause and menopause and seeking support for their journey. I invite you to speak up when a media outlet gets it wrong; it's the only way we're going to be able to reframe menopause from being something negative into being something worth celebrating. Let's call on advertisers and media to discard some of the outdated language they are using, because the way we've been thinking about menopause has actually been ruining our ability to enjoy it!

YOU Are Your Own Best Health Advocate

I'm going to begin this chapter with suggestions for having a conversation about perimenopause with your doctor, because I wrote an ebook about that a couple of years ago. These suggestions are transferable regardless of what health professional you are talking to.

However, let's get one thing clear. If you are reading this and saying to yourself "Why do I need to see a doctor?" that is absolutely okay! Menopause and perimenopause do not require treatments or cures, even though some product developers have led us to believe otherwise. Approximately 20% of women sail through perimenopause without any disruptive experiences. Another 20% have their worlds turned upside-down and the remaining 60% of women have experiences that are occasionally annoying or inconvenient. I hope you are a member of the smooth sailing club. And if not, then I also want you to know this:

1. Experiences related to midlife hormonal shifts are real.
2. You do not have to suck it up.
3. If one health care provider dismisses your experiences or tells you "you're not there yet," you have other options.

The experiences that are often associated with hormone fluctuations are frustrating, because they are most often the ones we dismiss the most ("we" being women). Particularly in our mid-thirties and throughout our forties, many of us are not really sure if we're dealing with perimenopause or symptoms of being stressed out due to our kids, work, marriage, or life in general.

Frustration grows when you add in the common misconception that menopause (and therefore any common experiences associated with it) do not start until you're fifty. This is completely incorrect!

So, when should you consult your doctor or seek out the advice of a midlife health expert? Often, women tend to put nuances in our health—whether slight or severe—on the back burner. However, not investigating these changes can mean overlooking something more serious that might be going on. You should always rule anything serious out; it's better to be safe than sorry.

The Menopause Book by Pat Wingert and Barbara Kantrowitz offers the following as a guideline for when you should see a doctor concerning symptoms possibly related to fluctuating hormones, midlife, and/or menopause and perimenopause:

- Irregular cycles
- Very heavy bleeding with clots, or periods that last more than a week
- Frequent spotting between periods
- Bleeding with pain or fever
- Blood in your urine
- Abrupt cessation of periods
- Symptoms that are interfering with your ability to function (hot flashes, night sweats, erratic bleeding)
- A missed period that could indicate pregnancy
- Any bleeding that occurs after one year of no menstrual periods
- Painful or swollen breasts
- Vaginal dryness/pain during intercourse
- Urinary problems/incontinence
- More than one panic attack
- A general sense of unhappiness or a persistent negative mood

- Inability to experience pleasure or to enjoy the things you used to do
- Constant worrying
- Chronic anxiety
- Obsessive thoughts or compulsive actions that you can't control
- Suicidal thoughts or paranoia
- Extreme fatigue, wired-but-tired, and/or sleep changes such as insomnia, inability to stay asleep, or oversleeping
- Significant weight changes
- Memory lapses that make it difficult for you to function normally
- Profound difficulty reading, writing, or speaking
- Anger or rage
- Itchy or restless legs
- Changes to skin and hair or hair loss
- Family history of thyroid problems

If you look back on my story about talking to my doctor about menopause, you'll realize that everything I've learned about preparing for a doctor's visit, I learned by *not* preparing for my doctor's visit. Thankfully, I've gained a few tips since then by reading books, interviewing health care professionals, and yes, even from searching the internet.

When it comes to your health, I encourage you to build a midlife health team—and for you to be captain of that team! You are the best person to be in the driver's seat. My hope is that women will be open to all of the options available to them: GP, naturopath, gynaecologist, doctor of natural medicine, registered nurse/nurse practitioner, registered dietitian, acupuncturist, chiropractor, yoga, energy therapy, massage therapy, Reiki, meditation coach, counsellor, laser therapy, reflexology, aromatherapy/essential oil therapy, fitness trainer, hypnotherapist, infrared sauna, vitamins and supplements, and even your local farmer's market.

I've chosen to treat my available options like a buffet—not closing any doors to any one avenue, yet creating a combination that works for me in this life phase. You might choose to blend traditional medicine with more holistic approaches. It may be possible to work with your doctor but also get support from a nutritionist, acupuncturist, therapist, or health coach. I see a family doctor for some things, a naturopath for others, and I try to round out those choices by paying attention to how I eat, move, and sleep. I also read a lot of health information. And always remember, the most important person on your health care team is you! If something doesn't sit well with you, trust yourself to speak up and voice your concerns.

Embracing the value of your primary care doctor and/or naturopathic doctor for continuity of care, preventative and reactive health measures, and regular testing such as Pap smears and mammograms is a key ingredient to midlife health. It's important, if possible, to choose someone you like and trust, which means familiarizing yourself with how your doctor was trained, what options he/she has in their toolkit, and how their particular modality or practice supports women in midlife transition. If you're unsure about someone's credentials, ask about them when booking the appointment. I say this because it's important to understand that not all naturopaths are hormone balance experts, but many are; not all doctors are trained or have expertise in perimenopause transition, but some are; and so on.

Here are a few tips on getting ready to crack open the conversation with your doctor/health care professional.

Be Informed

In medicine, as with many things in life, knowledge is power—and it's up to you to know your own medical history. Very few of us have had the luxury of having a single family doctor throughout our life who knows our history and has it all documented for review. Before your appointment, gather as much information as you can from the past five years, including your medical records. You have a right to your files, though there may be a fee to retrieve them. These records will help you establish a baseline, a history, and might avoid unnecessary repeat testing.

Start by talking to your mom, and to your sisters if possible. Get their history as well, especially around menopause and perimenopause. At what age did they first start noticing changes in their period? How old were they when they had their last period? What was their experience like, and how did they manage? There is no guarantee that your experience will be anything like your mom's or your sisters'; however, I believe it's still worth knowing.

Track Your Own Experiences

Health care professionals are scientists and will appreciate having visual evidence to support your story. You can use an app or a tracking chart. You should track your experiences for at least a month (or more); this will help your health care provider find solutions that are right for you.

Be Focused and Clear

When it comes time to book your appointment, make your discussion the only reason for the visit. Say, "I'd like to talk about perimenopause during this appointment—specifically about [any challenges or questions you might have]."

Perimenopause is not simple, so give it the attention and space it deserves. Don't tack it on to the end of an unrelated visit like I did—although the end of a visit may be a good time to open the discussion by saying you'd like *another* appointment specifically to have this conversation. Help your doctor more effectively plan the visit so that your needs are met without falling too far behind schedule. If they schedule ten-minute appointments, then giving them (or their staff) advance warning that you may need a longer appointment will make life easier for everyone.

When the appointment starts, advise your doctor at the beginning that you have questions—many of us don't have any idea how much time is actually scheduled with the doctor, and they're often running behind. If you're twenty minutes into your fifteen-minute appointment and you unexpectedly pull out a list of ten questions, he/she is going to have a hard time giving your questions the focus they deserve without upsetting other patients, the schedule—and you.

Be Open

We all have biases. It's only natural to have beliefs about how the world works—some ingrained in us by our families growing up, some newly acquired. There are beliefs like "pharmaceuticals are just looking to make money by calling everything a disease" to "alternative health care doctors are quacks," and everything in between.

Understand your own biases and be open to challenging how you think. Recognize and keep in mind that your doctor also has his or her own point of view and beliefs. It's so important that you are both speaking the same language. You need to have a common ground in the discussion where definitions are agreed upon and philosophies, biases, and viewpoints are on the table.

Not all doctors are hormone balance experts. If you happen to be consulting with someone who specializes in women's health, midlife health, or hormone health, fantastic! You must realize, though, that general practitioners can't be experts in everything, and they typically receive no more than an hour of training on this subject in medical school. They are, however, trained to respond to the symptoms you present. So, if you present as depressed or sleep-deprived, then they have medicinal ways to address and treat this. It helps to know in advance how you want to discuss prescription options, for example, and whether or not it is going to be the right solution for you.

Be Respectful

Give your doctor the same respect and attentiveness you expect to receive. Be on time for your appointment and understand that they have other patients to see, and that the conversation may have to continue over another appointment. Also, turn off your mobile device.

Be Empowered

Accept responsibility for your health and become a proactive partner in your own health care. You have a role to play, and it's not as a spectator. You may not be a doctor, but you are an expert in your own body and what you've been experiencing. Your job is to communicate that effectively, and to actively manage your health. The truth is, empowered patients are a relief to doctors, because doctors are problem solvers; they want to do a great job, but they can only do so when and if their patients meet them half way.

Stop worrying if you will offend your doctor; your health is far too important to not speak up! Your silence could also be perceived as understanding the test results or treatment options that are being explained. It's okay to be assertive. Speak your mind, and say what you have to say with authority. Don't let your doctor interrupt you or steamroll you. Say "no" when you don't agree. Be willing to question what your doctor says (respectfully, of course).

In the same vein, be careful not to make insensitive demands, such as "You've got to fix this," "Nothing you suggest ever works," or "I'm not leaving here until you agree to XYZ!" There is a distinct line between empowered and acting entitled.

Be Aware

Have you ever walked into a doctor's appointment with pressing health questions, and then forgot? Or, perhaps you felt rushed—or even too embarrassed to ask the questions once you were face-to-face?

There are a few interesting dynamics you should be aware of before you go to your appointment. There is something called productivity pressure—that's when your doctor stands up and puts his hand on the door handle, sending the message that he is busy and your time is done. Respect the length of time you have with the doctor, but don't hesitate to request a follow-up appointment to continue the conversation. Then, before you drive home, write down some notes about what you already discussed and what your next questions are. That way, you can start the next appointment with a recap for your doctor's benefit and keep the conversation rolling.

Also, something that has happened to me on more than one occasion is white coat syndrome—this is when patients who are confident, looking forward to their appointment, and know exactly what they want to discuss suddenly clam up or forget what they wanted to say once they're in front of their doctor. That's why writing down your questions is so important.

Avoid victim speak and blaming. Don't show up as a victim of bad luck or bad genes, or blame everything on your husband and/or kids. Accept responsibility for your circumstances, and for leading your health care provider to find solutions that will work for you. Show up as a proactive advocate willing to participate in your health, and your doctor will be more inclined to listen.

Be Supported

If you are concerned about getting confused or remembering all the instructions, or worry about standing your ground, bring support—your husband or partner, or maybe a girlfriend. Having a second set of eyes and ears can make a big difference as it's easy to feel overwhelmed when having these discussions, particularly if it's your first time cracking open this conversation, your first visit to a new physician, or you're already feeling overwhelmed in your day-to-day life. Be sure to tell your supporter what their role is in advance and give them a copy of your questions. They might think of other questions or ask clarifiying questions during the appointment that you would never have thought of. Be sure to introduce them (and their role) to your doctor at the beginning of the appointment.

Practice Telling Your Story

Doctors should know how to take a good history. Medical students devote a ton of time in medical school to mastering this skill, but depending on the circumstances (such as the length of your relationship with doctor or the complexity of situation) it may become your job to assist them. Make notes. Practice telling your story, and imagine being on the receiving end of your story and interpreting the situation. Don't be shy to tell your doctor what you think is going on—they've heard it all! Focus on telling your story as if you were speaking with a relative or a friend.

Dr. Leana Wen, author of *When Doctors Don't Listen*, offers the following tips for telling your story.

Tip #1: Start at the beginning and proceed chronologically. It helps the doctor to understand your story if you tell it in chronological order. For example: "I've been married for twenty-five years and my husband and I have always enjoyed a healthy sex life. Then about a year ago, I noticed I no longer had any desire for sex. And six months ago, I realized that vaginal dryness was also getting in the way. It's now been a year since we've been intimate, and this has dramatically affected my relationship, not to mention my own self-esteem and well-being."

Tip #2: Use concepts such as timing, pace, onset of symptoms,

severity, and changes over time to tell a stronger story. For example: "Having two small children, I was used to waking up in the middle of the night. But, I could always manage to get back to sleep, and I don't recall ever feeling overly sleep deprived. For the last six months, no matter what time I go to bed, I wake up at 3:00 a.m. and I can never seem to get back to sleep. It's affecting my ability to work, to care for my family, and to function at the level I am accustomed to."

Tip #3: Draw it out. Track your symptoms and plot them on a graph. The horizontal axis can be any time interval you choose (day-to-day, week-to-week, or month-to-month, depending on your symptoms). The vertical axis is your level of severity. Record a number on a scale of one to ten, with one being minimal and ten being the worst. If there are two or more symptoms of concern, you can plot them alongside each other.

Tip #4: Describe how your symptoms/current experiences are impacting your life. Your doctor may ask you to quantify your symptoms in an objective way. Provide an answer, but also expand on it. Telling your doctor that you've been experiencing anxiety attacks and needing to leave work early, or that you're having difficulty performing day-to-day chores, will be more helpful than simply describing your depression as being a seven out of ten. Also, explaining the impact on your daily life gives your doctor a window to who you are and improves your chances of the doctor making the right diagnosis.

Tip #5: If something about your experiences surprised you, emphasize it. Share both your expectations and your surprises. For example: "I'm getting used to having irregular periods. However, the bleeding has become so heavy and erratic—it has really caught me off guard, and I can barely leave the house. This has never happened before!" Relating what's surprising to you will help make sure the doctor pays attention to this part and address it. And who knows; it might surprise your doctor too, and completely change his or her thought process.

Tip #6: If there is a diagnosis that you are particularly concerned about, let your doctor know up front. If you're worried about a brain tumor, being told to take Advil might not be the answer you're looking for. If you are concerned about seeming too presumptuous, you can always say something like, "Look, I'm not a doctor or anything, but I have a cousin who had these similar headaches and she ended up being diagnosed with cancer. Should I be worried?" Sharing your fears can help your doctor consider a wider list of possibilities, and can also potentially alleviate your concerns.

Tip #7: Write it down. Your story may be long and winding, with twists and turns that aren't necessarily straightforward. To help make sure the important parts of the story aren't left out, use a symptom tracker and write down your story. If you are experiencing symptoms over a number of months, it might help to keep a journal. You can use the journal to keep track of other aspects of your daily life (activities, eating habits, sleep patterns, treatments you've tried and what you're currently taking, and more) to the extent that you think they may relate to your symptoms. This information can be incredibly helpful in leading you and your doctor to the best solution for you.

Second Opinions

We live in a society where we are taught to respect professionals, be polite, and accept medical opinion as gospel. However, while many physicians understand perimenopause, there are some who do not.

Not wanting to offend or be demanding is okay. What's not okay is to accept treatment, surgery, or care that doesn't fit with your values, or your gut. In those cases, you should explore a second (or third, or fourth) opinion, and your doctor will hopefully welcome and endorse it—if not, then are you really consulting the right health care provider in the first place? You should not leave a medical appointment feeling defeated or humiliated.

Seeking second opinions is actually not a common occurrence. This either tells us that most patients are pretty satisfied with the care their provider recommends, or that we are too shy, too busy, too overwhelmed, or maybe simply unaware that this is an option. It's your job to be your own best health advocate; you must be an informed patient and do what's best for you.

While seeking a second opinion is not common among patients, you may be surprised to learn how often medical professionals seek formal or informal second opinions from each other. Research results and new medical developments happen at such a rapid pace that physicians are in a state of continuous learning—sometimes via their own research or by attending conferences, but often it is by consulting with each other.

If you decide to get a second opinion, be sure to tell your doctor. Otherwise, it will be hard to get the records or test results that you'll need to communicate with other health care professionals. You can start the second opinion process by asking for a referral. If you're not confident in your physician's ability to help you address your concerns, ask them to refer you to an endocrinologist or someone who has more experience treating hormone imbalances.

Also, be up front with the second professional rather than waiting for their diagnosis to say, "But that's not what I was told by Dr. A!" You might begin with simply stating "I'm here to get a second opinion" or explaining the concerns you have with your first recommendation, such as saying, "My doctor said I need X, but I feel like he really didn't listen to me when I was describing my experience. I'm worried he's recommending X without hearing my whole story."

Be Prepared

The way we frame our thoughts around a doctor's appointment is quite interesting. For example, have you ever found yourself worrying about

what they might ask you—do you smoke, when was your last Pap, are you sexually active, how many drinks do you have per week?

It's time for a paradigm shift. It isn't about what *they* are going to ask *you*, it's about what *you* will ask *them*. A 2012 study in the Journal of Health Affairs states that people don't ask their health care providers questions for fear being perceived as difficult, although that might be a generational thing—I know my parents would have never thought to question or challenge their doctors. What if you were to reframe your thinking around your doctor-patient relationship? You expect your doctor to do his/her job; it is *your* job to show up and be prepared. Make a list of questions and take it with you, so you can be sure that your concerns are addressed.

The kinds of questions you ask your doctor will vary depending on whether you are inquiring about what changes you could experience in the coming years, or if you've been dealing with symptoms for some time. Prepare for your appointment by getting informed, tracking your experiences and organizing the questions that pertain to your personal situation.

You may also prioritize your questions according to how much time is allotted for your appointment so you can get the most pressing concerns addressed first.

Here is a list of questions around perimenopause or menopause that you may consider asking your doctor or other health care provider. Remember to write your questions down before you go!

- Is this common?
- Could my experiences be caused by a condition other than perimenopause?
- If my experiences are interfering with my ability to function at the level I am used to, or to get a good night's sleep, do they warrant treatment?
- Do I still need birth control?

- Am I now at a higher risk for heart disease, osteoporosis, or other conditions?
- What do you recommend I have checked so I have a baseline going forward?
- What tests do you recommend?
- What are the benefits of testing blood versus saliva versus urine?
- Should I be checking my:
    - thyroid?
    - cholesterol?
    - blood pressure?
    - bone density?
- What are you prescribing?
    - Is it the lowest dose possible?
    - What are the known side effects?
    - Are there any other options we can consider?
    - How might it interact with other things I'm taking (drugs, vitamins, herbs)?
    - How long do you recommend we try this approach, and what is the exit strategy?
    - Where can I get more info?
- What are the pros and cons to hormone therapy?
- What is your recommended protocol (straight to hormone therapy, or try other approaches first)?
- Can you please explain your particular recommendations around hormone therapy? Who is it right for? How long should a woman stay on it? How can I find out more before making my decision?
- Can you explain the difference between synthetic hormones and bioidentical hormones?
- How do you decide between methods such as oral, gel, or patch, and between over-the-counter versus prescription medications?

- Are there health and lifestyle recommendations that might address these symptoms such as alcohol, caffeine, diet, exercise, or vitamin supplements?
- What can you tell me about the benefits of yoga, acupuncture, and herbal remedies?
- What do I need to know about the placebo effect, and is there a way this might help me?

Write your own specific questions here:

The Invisible Backpack

When I started out to write this book, I assumed it would be like most other projects I've tackled in my career. Do this, then this, then this and boom, I'd have a book. And then, the events of this chapter happened.

This chapter took almost an entire year to unfold. Here's what happened in a nutshell: I acted like I was invincible, I didn't walk my own talk, and I ended up with a mental illness diagnosis—which just might have been the blessing I'd been waiting on.

More on that in a minute.

First, I'd like to share with you an article I wrote in January of 2017 for my website, commemorating #BellLetsTalkDay in Canada. I remember the feeling as I hit the send button. I wasn't being completely overt, but I knew that I was in a space in my life where I needed some attention and support. Four weeks later, I found myself sitting in my naturopath's office hearing her say "post traumatic stress disorder," and a few days later, after answering what seemed like seven simple questions, I heard my family doctor utter the word "bipolar." Here is the article, titled "My Invisible Backpack":

> Today is Bell Let's Talk Day in Canada—a chance for all of us to crack open the conversation on mental health, create a stigma-free society, and raise funds for critical mental health and wellness programs and services.

As I was pouring over all the great resource materials Bell has created, I couldn't help but draw some obvious parallels between perimenopause and menopause (topics I talk about every day) and mental health (a topic I'm not afraid to discuss, yet one I tend to only crack open when absolutely necessary). Here are seven ways navigating MENTAL HEALTH is like navigating MENOPAUSE:

1. BOTH MAKE US LIE: Cultural myths, generational stereotypes, stigma, fear of what people will think... whatever the reason, both mental health and menopause make us lie; they can make us say we're "fine" when we are not.
2. BOTH NEED A RE-BRAND: Branding, if you don't know, is defined as what others say about you when you are not in the room. It commonly refers to corporate brands, but branding also refers to the "bad rap" or outdated reputation that continues to swirl around both mental health and menopause. If you say mental health or menopause, people often assume they know exactly what you are talking about–except, more often than not, they are drawing upon old myths, misconceptions, outdated images and information, and negative stereotypes.
3. BOTH ARE COMPLEX AND SURROUNDED WITH PROMISES OF CURES: What if we replaced words like "cure" with "manage" or "navigate"? Rather than continuing to mask and suppress our experiences, what if we were to start recognizing these journeys as OPPORTUNITIES to stop and figure out what's up in life; to enhance how well we eat, move, and sleep; to introduce new or increased stress management protocols; to practice more self love?
4. BOTH ARE MISUNDERSTOOD: Depression is

not the same as sadness, and menopause is not equal to suffering.

5. BOTH ARE PART OF THE HUMAN EXPERIENCE: Society often wants to compartmentalize us, placing us in categories like "she has a mental illness" and "she does not." What if we reframe this so that mental health is a spectrum (a very important spectrum!) rather than an isolated circumstance? For many, it's more like a dial that gets turned up or turned down at various points in our lives. What if we repositioned it as part of the human experience? Something everyone needs to know about, know how to talk about, and most importantly, know how to navigate—for themselves, and for their loved ones? The same is true for the perimenopause-to-menopause journey.
6. THE STRUGGLE IS REAL, THE EXPERIENCE IS UNIQUE FOR EVERYONE, AND THERE IS A MAGIC WAND AFTER ALL: If I've learned anything over these past few years managing the Menopause Chicks community, it's that there are a million combinations of what's right and wrong, and what works and doesn't work, but the one common ground where we all seem to land is how good it feels to be validated. Feeling understood and validated is the magic—be it mental health, menopause, or any other situation that calls for compassion.
7. REACHING OUT IS THE OPPOSITE OF STIGMA: As Prince Harry said, "I just needed someone to listen." If we truly want to eradicate the stigma associated with mental health and menopause, more of us need to reach out. As I've learned with the Menopause Chicks Private Online Community, reaching out for help—or even just finding a caring ear—moves us away from naiveness, avoidance, and the suppression of what is real. Instead, it moves us closer

to awareness, education, compassion, understanding, and conversation.

For many years now, I have referred to my own challenges with anxiety, depression, and brain fog as "my invisible backpack"; it's the thing I carry everywhere that nobody can see.

At times, I even make up imaginary conversations where I invite people close to me to peek inside the backpack. I let them know it's okay if they've never noticed it before, because I have worked very hard to camouflage it. It's taken me a good long while to admit I even have a backpack, but now I'm growing more comfortable showing it to people.

I tell them about how I carry it everywhere. About how some days it's light and I can forget it's even there, and other days it can get really heavy. I share how tired it makes me to carry this load around with me everywhere I go.

Once upon a time, I was probably worried about what people would think of me if I confessed to having anxiety and feelings of depression. The charade of pretending to be okay would be over. The truth would be out: I do not have all of my shit together. However, what I've learned is that everyone is carrying something, and it is almost always invisible until we talk about it. Most people smile and let me know that I am not alone. Many people reply with a simple "me too."

I want to challenge all of us to rethink our perceptions of what mental illness is and looks like—of what health is and looks like. Google may tell us it's a dark picture of a woman looking sad and holding her head in her hands, but I'm here to tell you it might also look like a smiling, high-functioning, responsible adult. Do I "have" post-traumatic stress disorder, as my naturopath questioned, or do I "have" bipolar disorder, as the seven-question quiz I took suggested? Or, had I forgotten to take care of myself for a good, long time, resulting in "my dial" getting turned a little too far down the spectrum toward mental illness? I don't know the definitive answer to this. What I do know is that my health team prescribed exercise and counselling, and I took them up on those recommendations. Mental health is a wide spectrum. It is—like perimenopause, menopause and post-menopause—part of the human experience. And by that, I mean it is meant to be experienced.

Let's not let past stigmas and stereotypes dictate our futures or prevent us from recognizing what people may be carrying. If you need some words today, try "I hear you," "I see you," and "you are not alone."

So, back to feeling and acting invinsible…

When I stepped onto the TedxGastownWomen stage in October 2016 with a big, beautiful butterfly image behind me, I felt as if I had the world by the tail. I was forty-nine, and I had reached and celebrated menopause. I was hashtagging everything with #ilovemidlife, and I was positive that I was a fully-grown butterfly, ready to rock fifty and beyond.

So what did I do?

I became completely enthralled in my new entrepreneurial adventure. I stopped exercising, I stopped going to yoga, I stopped putting my own name at the top of my to-do list, and I stopped taking my hormone therapy. DO NOT DO WHAT I DID! I repeat, do not start, stop, or adjust dosages of any prescription without the guidance of your health care professional.

What followed was a few months of feeling okay. Then, all the same issues began to resurface—the brain fog, anxiety, depression, and sleep deprivation—and it spilled over into my work and relationships like hot lava from a smoldering volcano. And even though I was in the middle of it, I seemed incapable of doing anything to stop it.

Why do we assume the journey to become a butterfly is easy? I mean, the butterfly literally turns itself inside out and has to trust that it isn't dying in the process. If you look at the science diagrams of a butterfly's metamorphosis, you'll notice there are at least six to seven stages illustrated—and the final three to four all look like butterflies. It doesn't go from chrysalis to fully-grown butterfly in one flash step. It's a process; a concept that I clearly missed, as I now know what it feels like to literally turn myself inside out and trust that I'm not dying. And every day, I'm grateful for the process, because it brought me back here to this process of writing and planning next steps for Menopause Chicks and delivering this book to you.

So, it's natural to ask the questions: do I have a mental illness? Are my experiences hormonal? The answers are certainly ambiguous to me. And that's okay. Life—and certainly managing our midlife health—is not black-and-white. I can call it a spectrum. I can call it a Rubik's cube. The thing I have learned the most through my journey is the importance of making myself a priority, listening to what my mind and body are telling me, and understanding that I am always changing, always learning, and always growing. Things are always better when I pay attention to myself, because what we focus on expands.

My midlife health team now consists of my naturopath, family doctor, counsellor, and pharmacist. My midlife plan includes regular massages, acupuncture when I can, daily adrenal support, hormone therapy (bi-est and progesterone), iron, omega-3s, magnesium, iodine, and vitamins B, C, and D. I also spend time in counselling and take part in meditation. Every day, I try to include exercise, a healthy dose of determination, forgiveness and self-talk, plus lots of check-ins with my sister, dear friends, and loved ones.

The other thing this recent journey reminded me of was the power of being vulnerable, and the overwhelming love and support that can be yours when you do. I've been practicing vulnerability, and now whenever I say mokitas like "money challenges" or "my marriage has been bumpy" or "I have been taking care of my mental health" to a friend or a business colleague or a health professional, I am guaranteed to be met with a kind smile and an "Oh ya, me too. You are not alone."

This is validation, and connection.

"You are not alone" are the four words I write the most to Menopause Chicks in our private online community, and the four words that have empowered me to navigate my own midlife health journey with confidence and ease.

The Graduation Party

Now, if you think getting shut down at a cocktail party for saying the word "menopause" is too much, imagine the reactions I got in 2016 when I told people I was actually going to throw myself a party to commemorate the one year anniversary of my last period!

It's not an occasion many (any?) of us celebrate, but this was one of my various attempts to get women—and men—talking about menopause as a normal part of life. And since menopause only comes along once in a lifetime, I knew I had to go for it! The invitation went like this:

HAPPY MENOPAUSE TO ME!
HAPPY MENOPAUSE TO ME!
Happy Menopause Dear Shirley. Happy Menopause to Me!

That's right, my twelve months are up, and I'm getting ready to celebrate with Canadian rockstar Bif Naked!

I remember it like it was yesterday. I was away at a spa retreat with a few of my BFFs. You may find this surprising, but I am not fond of talking about bodily functions (says the girl who started a website about menopause!).

So there I was, coming home from a lovely dinner, working up the courage to tell my friends, "Hey girls! I haven't had a period for ten months. That's right. In just two more months, I'm going to invent a martini and have a party! I want to demystify perimenopause and menopause and really help women find the journey that's right for them. What better way to do that than to celebrate my own menopause!"

That night, I got my period. In the hotel room. Totally unexpected. Totally unprepared.

A part of me thought I ought to be happy that I "wasn't there yet." But I was crushed, because, you know...martinis!

For the next few months, my period was textbook-regular. And then the countdown (party planning!) began AGAIN.

As I write this note to you, I am forty-nine years old and just days away from celebrating...you guessed it...MY MENOPAUSE.

Cue the confetti. Shake that martini. I'm having an online party to celebrate. It's an online soiree where smart women (and some smart men too!) of all ages will be joining me to get more clarity, validation, and inspiration to live a happy, healthy midlife!

On April 19, 2016, at age forty-nine, I did host my party. I celebrated reaching the milestone of menopause and encouraged hundreds of my online guests to learn more about their own journey, or the journey of their loved ones, as they moved from perimenopause to menopause and beyond.

Okay, I admit, a party to celebrate one's menopause milestone may seem a bit far-fetched or unusual. You don't need to host a party if that's not your thing. It's not the concept of the party that is important, it is the celebratory aspect; the reframing of menopause that is key. Let's continue to celebrate this milestone so we ignite a paradigm shift. Let's reframe menopause from something that is regarded as mostly negative into a life phase that is honoured, respected, and celebrated.

I was joined at my party by Vancouver-based rock star and cancer survivor Bif Naked, who had her ovaries removed at age thirty-seven. She came to share her perspective on celebrating menopause, an interview I had manifested for a little more than a year. You see, in March 2015, Bif wrote an article for the Globe & Mail newspaper about her experience with menopause, which I devoured. Even though our journeys to menopause were very different (hers being surgical, and mine natural), I literally printed the article off and hugged the paper it was printed on before pinning it on my bulletin board. I promised myself that I would follow her advice as I counted down the months to menopause. That same week I saw Bif in a television interview with Jody Vance, encouraging all women to have a party to celebrate their menopause milestone. Yes, a party! I was in.

The article was titled "Learning to Love Menopause," and there was a phrase in the article that jumped off the page for me: **"I am here to tell you these myths are all wrong. Menopause is actually pretty cool."**

In the rest of the article, she talked about how she learned very little about menopause growing up. Her grandmother and mother were apprehensive and shy toward the topic, and almost considered it impolite to discuss hot flashes, mood swings, weight gain, or body rashes. Bif learned about these notorious menopause experiences probably in much the same way you or I did—through whispers and secrets, public rumour, and of course, the media.

I loved how Bif called herself an expert on menopause, thanks to getting thrown into this phase at thirty-seven. Imagine how different our health care system and our approach to health might be if we all thought of ourselves as our own best experts!

She referenced being cold for most of her life, "So when I started experiencing hot flashes they were a welcome phenomenon for a teeth-chattering-in-the-sunshine skinny little vegan singer like myself. I loved it!" And then she went on to share her personal list of the benefits of menopause, from saving money when you kiss your tampons away, to writing songs at 3:00 a.m. when you can't sleep, to getting bigger breasts and a chance to embrace your changing body, your femaleness, and the gifts of your gender. Again, these benefits are not shared so everyone would agree with her list, but rather to bravely point out that if we can reframe how we think about midlife transition, we can reframe our experience in a positive way.

In her words, "If this is the change-of-life, I say make mine a change for the better!...I am the girl who will always, come hell or hot flashes, find the bright side and the silver lining."

It was that article that got Bif to my menopause party. And now, before I give you my next invitation, I have a question for you.

What do you think of when I say menopause? Old? Hot? Tired? The beginning of the end? Women will often give me an even longer list that includes things like irregular periods, heavy bleeding, loss of libido, memory loss, less hair where they want it and more hair where they don't, depression, anxiety, and even bouts of rage.

But some may hear the word "menopause" and think wise, confident, beautiful, and free. Or, simply, no big deal.

If that's the case, then we definitely have a gap.

I believe the way we think of menopause is ruining our ability to enjoy it. As people like Bif Naked are pointing out, we have a tendency to take on the negative views of society and advertisers and stop there, without contemplating any of the potential positives.

What if, instead of thinking of menopause as the beginning of the end, we thought of it simply as the beginning?

This ah-ha moment came to me shortly after I started my website. A young reporter called me—I knew she must be twenty-something based on how she described the perimenopause experiences of her mother and aunt.

I tried to help her with the article she was writing by launching into everything I had been learning about perimenopause and menopause. I started to explain to her how menopause is just one day, and on average occurs around 51.2 years of age; that perimenopause is the five to fifteen years of hormone fluctuations leading up to menopause, and perimenopause can begin as early as your mid-to-late thirties.

I was just about to tell her how there is very little research on perimenopause—in fact, the term perimenopause wasn't even coined until the 1990's. "So," I said, "if your grandmother said she was 'going through menopause,' she likely meant 'going through perimenopause!'"

As I was telling her all of this, the young reporter interrupted me and said, **"Wow. You must be the SMARTEST you've ever been!"**

I was stunned! Nobody had ever really said anything like that to me before, and while I had read a lot about perimenopause, there was no indication it would make me smarter! Then, I considered her words. Maybe she was right. I am smart, and wiser than I used to be, and more confident too.

If I can learn to park the inconvenient experiences of perimenopause over to the side, I realize that midlife shines a big, bright spotlight on who I am and what I want in my life. It's a time when self-care becomes a priority, and when my own name is at the top of my to-do list!

That reporter gave me an amazing gift that day. She inspired me not to miss any part of this beautiful unfolding.

And now, my invitation to you: will you help me write a new script for menopause? Can we reframe it so we learn how to navigate any challenges **AND** celebrate the positives too? And when we close the gap—when we are intentional with our positive word choice—just imagine how women will *look forward to midlife*! And that's a good thing, because if we plan to live to be 100, we will spend half of our lives on the other side of this important milestone.

Menopause is not a disease or something that needs to be "fixed." It should not be a mokita or an elephant in the room, a topic only discussed in hushed tones and private conversations.

Join me in cracking open the conversation and helping women (and men) of all ages learn to celebrate menopause.

Part II

How to Build Your Own Midlife Health Team

Introduction to Part II

When I started down this journey to discover all of the best perimenopause information I can find, the lines that divided the camps between traditional/mainstream/conventional medicine and more preventative/holistic/natural medicine were very distinct. There were unwritten rules about what you could talk about with whom.

We are now seeing evidence of a less-defined line between the two; more cross-over, greater respect, and more and more examples of integrated health clinics and patient-centric, integrated approaches to health care. There are now examples of naturopathic clinics within hospitals, and some Canadian naturopaths have been granted permission to prescribe some drugs and order lab tests (although this varies province to province).

Why is this important? I believe women need more choices—choices that not only address the particular experience (symptom), but also the underlying root cause. With more collaboration between health professionals comes more flexibility in treatment, more options becoming available, and more knowledge on how each modality can benefit you.

It's important for you to know where your personal preferences lie so you know which path to pursue first, which services are covered by your health care plan, and what you need to budget for. Having a firm grasp on your desired approach will hopefully save you time, money, and frustration in the long run.

It's time now for this book to switch gears, and for me to pass the torch to my phenomenal co-authors. Presented in alphabetical order by last name, each co-author will give you insight into their own specialty and how it can be used to support you through your perimenopause and menopause experiences. They will expand even more on the information you have learned throughout this book, adding in their own specialized knowledge to provide you with in-depth information on each topic.

To give you even further insights on how these different modalities can impact your perimenopause-to-menopause journey, many have included case studies that show how their practice is applied to real-life situations or examples of treatments or approaches they use.

Be sure to read each co-author's biography beginning on page 240.

Get ready to feel empowered to build your own midlife team.

Liz Applegate, Personal Life Coach

If there were a one-word theme that appeared most often with my clients over forty, it would be "change."

Not only is there the desire for change, but life itself seems to bring about change on its own. There are physical changes taking place, and there are also changes in how we see the world around us, and even how the world sees us.

Physically, our bodies are changing. The bathroom mirror reflects crow's feet and sun damage. Our hormones are fluctuating, which affects our menstrual cycle, sleep, weight, and mood. Even our digestion and food intolerances can be thrown off.

The roles we play in our daily lives can also be changing. If we have children, we begin to wonder about our new role as mom as they begin graduating high school. Careers can now seem lackluster as goals of climbing the corporate ladder and achieving a fancy title no longer fulfill us. We dream of travelling and experiencing something new. We crave a life of purpose and meaning.

Change can be happening in our relationships too. Friendships are looked at carefully. Marriages are viewed with a new perspective that can make them seem stifling. Often, through raising children, partners have forgotten who they are as a couple. We question if our partner even knows who we are; but, we can often feel as if we don't even know ourselves at this stage in life.

We realize that we can no longer relate to characters in movies and television shows. Doors are no longer held open for us the way they once were. How in the world are we supposed to dress now?

When all of these changes and realizations collide, it can feel like a rug has been pulled out from us. We can be left asking ourselves, "Who am I in these 'middle years' of life?"

This was the question that I asked myself in my mid-forties. It's one that I continue to work on now, both with myself and with the women who are my clients.

My Story

I like to joke that my forties were the red wine and chocolate phase of my life, but honestly it wasn't a joke—and it wasn't very funny at the time.

The challenges began at age thirty-nine, when I found myself a divorced mother of three sons. I was once told that getting a divorce was similar to taking a deck of cards, throwing it up into the air, and then trying to choose and catch the most important cards. Little did I know this was the beginning of many times when I would have to decide what was important.

If I back my story up just a few years to my mid-thirties, I realize now that I had been experiencing perimenopause for some time. Heavy periods that could last up to six weeks had me enduring uterine biopsies, two dilation and curettage (D & C) procedures, and even birth control, despite the fact I had a my "tubes tied" after the birth of my youngest son. I was experiencing mood swings and difficulty sleeping. I was given prescriptions to control anxiety and depression, and with all of this—and much that I didn't understand—I began to gain weight.

I didn't have the answers that I was so desperately seeking. Even after seeing four doctors in a three-year span, I had been told by all of them that I was simply getting older, and that my "condition" was something to get used to.

In all honesty, by the time I turned forty, I felt that my body had betrayed me.

For the next six years, there were not only the physical changes but also emotional challenges. My sons all graduated high school and were headed to college, and I began questioning my role as their mom. Who was I, now that my day-to-day interaction with them was no longer needed? What was my purpose in life now that I had raised these three independent young men who were flying the nest quicker than my heart was ready for?

I shockingly lost friends in the divorce. I remarried, blended our families, changed careers, and experienced an emergency hysterectomy, which threw me into full-blown menopause. To say that I was questioning the life that I was living and the purpose that I now had was an understatement. The combination of my reality and the reality of what society was saying about this time in my life was purely shocking. I couldn't relate to the images of gray-haired women sitting in front of fans every time I searched the Internet for answers. I couldn't relate to the actresses being phased out of sexy, lively roles. I couldn't relate to feeling invisible, to being called "ma'am" instead of "miss," to no longer turning heads, to not knowing where to shop for clothes, let alone which department to shop in. Wasn't there something between low-cut-slinky-after-hours and elastic-waist-frumpy?

The Defining Moment

When I was pregnant with my children, I carried around the mom-bible "What to Expect When You Are Expecting." I read it cover to cover and reread it as needed with each pregnancy. Once I hit forty, though, I found minimal resources and very few positive voices. I once asked my gynaecologist in his office, surrounded by photos of young mothers and powdery-fresh newborns, where all of the books on "What to Expect When You Reach Midlife" were. Sadly, there wasn't an answer, and I knew that I had crossed into a new stage of my life without a map or even acceptable road signs.

It was at that moment that I realized it was time to actively seek out the information and support I was looking for, and to become part of a much-needed voice for other women. It was time that I found real change that would catapult me into living my best midlife, and to partner with women to help them do the same.

This is where my clients are too: wondering if this is all there is, and not happy for it to be so. They are seeking desired changes, although often they know how to make the changes—they just have to own what needs to happen and move through the uncomfortable places of change. Because let's face it, if change was easy, most of life's problems would be a breeze. And this where a life coach can help.

Life Coaching Explained

Life coaching is a relatively new form of support and often gets confused with therapy. I recently learned a great analogy to use when explaining coaching and counselling: a person may see a personal trainer to work certain muscles of the body so they can reach their desired goals, but the same person may also see a physical therapist to repair certain muscles that are weakened and need extra care to mend and heal. The same holds true for a life coach; we are the "personal trainers" for your life.

I work with my clients, who have a particular goal in mind. Maybe it's how to start that business they have always dreamed of, but now realize that it won't happen without some support and accountability. Maybe my client realizes that she doesn't know who she is during this time in her life—all of the changes that are taking place has her questioning her identity, and she doesn't want to settle for a life half-lived. I've helped clients change careers. I've helped clients be comfortable enough to take the dance class they have always wanted to take, or to the make art they always wanted to create, or to plan that solo trip to exotic places. And I've even worked with clients who were exploring their feelings about their marriage and if they wanted to continue with it.

My clients want to live their lives fully and realize that they need to take an active role in doing so. But it's through my own experience that I can also have my clients look at what is going on physically, at the "good girl rules" that are impacting where they are now, and at the ways they need to care for themselves while changes are taking place.

From Good Girl to Empowered Woman

No matter how strong our desire is, fear is what keeps us stuck. It's the running undercurrent of the choices we make and don't make. I'm not talking about the fear we experience from riding a roller coaster; I'm talking about the inner fears that we have a conversation with on a daily basis. It's the voice that is telling us we aren't good enough, smart enough, thin enough, young enough. These conversations are from our inner critic, or the "inner mean girl" as I like to call her. She's the bully that keeps us playing small, and I believe that she was given the parameters on how to work her damage when we were taught to be a "good girl" at a young age.

You know those rules, right? "Don't be so loud." "Don't ask so many questions." "Don't be bossy." "Don't be so emotional." "Children should be seen and not heard." It's what my coach calls "feminine conditioning."

Maybe these rules weren't meant to be damaging, but often we learned through these constant expectations that who we are isn't good enough. We learned to take up as small of a space as possible, and that means physically, emotionally, and mentally. It often meant that we put our wishes and dreams aside for the betterment of someone else. We disregarded the careers we dreamt of having. We believed that it was wrong to stand up for our beliefs, our ideas, and our dreams. We didn't ask for help out of fear of sounding needy. And we took what was offered to us, no matter how small, without expecting better. We've been taught that wanting more meant that we were selfish.

So, these rules have shaped and formed us from a young age. And here we are, in the middle years of our lives, still living by the rules that were laid out for us at age five, with an inner mean girl who reminds us when we get out of line. But what happens when we make this realization, and decide that our inner bully is just that—a voice from someone with limiting rules that want us to play small and be safe. We learn that it's okay to want better, and it's more than okay to stand up for those desires. And, despite the inner mean girl's best efforts, it's even okay to ask for help.

As a life coach, this is where the magic happens for my clients. When we can see where they are playing small and safely recognize how they are holding themselves back, it is the start of bravely rebuilding these identifying rules for ourselves as amazing women with unique life experiences. These women realize that those "maybe someday" dreams that have been ignored for far too long can be a reality; or, maybe they simply allow themselves to finally dream.

Every client I work with has a different journey and a different outcome they desire. I meet my clients where they are on their journey, but the beginning of each relationship begins with establishing a few practices that I share. These are common practices to come across when working with coaches, but what is different about my approach is that I recognize that the physiological experiences of perimenopause can be a factor in moving forward.

Getting Real to Make Positive Change

I couldn't just share my story and my philosophies without sharing one of my favourite exercises that I use when working with clients.

These simple daily practices can help you make progress in working toward a goal and recognize the area where you may not feel your best.

I recommend setting aside about an hour of uninterrupted time. Make a cup of your favourite tea or other beverage that signifies "special" to you. Put on soothing music. Grab a special notebook just for your exploration, along with a pen or pencil, and read and work through any of the prompts below. Just honouring this time begins the process of accepting who you are. Consider how often throughout our lives we rush from activity to activity and let the needs of others dictate your day. It's now time to reclaim your time and honour your desires.

A note about negative thoughts: chances are that you will have them while working on this exercise. After all, you are taking time for yourself, being honest, and openly examining how you want your life to look. Pay attention to places where the negative inner critic is showing up. Don't just push the comments away—get curious about them. Dedicate a page in your notebook just for this exploration. Write down what you are saying and then ask yourself about these thoughts. An example would be, "Why do you think this is a waste of time?"

Journal the thoughts that come up for you after you ask the questions below. Is this a place that your "good girl" rules are showing up? Is wanting better and more out of your life bringing up feelings of being selfish or ungrateful? It's important to pay attention to our inner dialogue and get curious as to where these thoughts come from, so we can reveal the places that are keeping us stuck.

Begin introducing "and" as you reframe your negative inner conversations. You can want better AND be grateful for what you have. You can be grieving time gone by AND still believe there are many happy memories to be made in the future.

Steps to Create Your Ultimate Day

Now we are going to create your Ideal Day Checklist, which means we need to get back to the basics. You will be doing some exploration of how to set up your day so you can feel your very best. This exercise will also have you looking at places that the experiences of perimenopause can be holding you back, and thus identifying the specific areas you need support around. This exercise takes into account the basics of daily living, but it also looks at our habits, both good and bad. Habits from when you were twenty may no longer apply to our current lives, yet many of us are still operating with those same habits that make up our lifestyle.

Take your time and consider the prompts below. Write them out and journal about each one when more thoughts come up around the subject.

- When have you felt the best physically? What were you eating and drinking? How much sleep were you getting? What supplements or medications were you taking?
- What meals have you had that left you feeling not well?
- What are your thoughts on movement and exercise?
- Do you practice meditation and/or prayer? Are you interested in exploring this?
- How much negativity are you allowing into your life? Think of people who drain your energy. Consider how the nightly news affects your mood. Think about how social media plays into your thoughts and if it's used as a form of escape.
- What makes you happy? Name the people, places, and activities. Go wild here—list everything! Indulge in happiness.
- Where can you be more generous? Giving of our time and love is just as important as giving our money.

- What fills your heart with gratitude? What are you thankful for? Name at least ten things, even if they seem small to you, like having the ability to read this page.
- What have you always wanted to learn how to do? Name as many things as you can think of.
- Imagine how you want your life to look in ten years. How do you look? What are you doing? How and where are you living? Dream, get creative, and describe yourself in full detail.

Putting It All together

Take a look at what you just explored and pull together a daily check list. Make the list as short or long as you wish; however, don't make it so long that it's stressful, and don't sell yourself short either. I have ten items on my list that I've grouped in headings.

Look at what's emerged as being important to you. Though this may seem overwhelming at first, over time this becomes a list of good habits to follow. It's something that you can remind yourself of each morning, and at the end of the day you can check in with it to see how well you have done and the results of your mindfulness. If you aren't feeling well or are unhappy, is there something on your list that you forgot that you can intentionally include tomorrow?

It's awareness. It's permission. It's a rinse-and-repeat situation that is different for us all.

This checklist is also a reminder to be mindful of your feelings and honour where you are on any particular day. It's a place to return to each day and make yourself a priority. Please read that again: this is a list to begin making yourself a priority. To plan out YOUR day to reflect what is important to YOU, what makes YOU happy, and the steps to start honouring who YOU are now, how far you've come, and your dreams for the future.

When I am feeling stressed and find that I'm playing into the "shoulds" of others, I need to remind myself to go back to the basics and see what I have let slip. Here is an example of my Ideal Day Checklist:

1. **Drink enough water.** For me, I feel best when I drink half of my weight in ounces.
2. **Be mindful of what I allow in and where I am showing up.** I need to pay attention to mindless social media scrolling and other self-numbing activities. Also, I need to be wary of people who I don't feel I can be myself with and who I consider "energy suckers."
3. **Get enough sleep.** I'm a natural night owl, but honestly, that was not serving me. It had become a habit, almost like an addiction, so this was an area that I discussed with my doctor. I was able to get a recommendation for a natural supplement that helps relax me and stay asleep. I also developed habits around my sleep. Most nights that means that I'm off computer/TV/iPad/iPhone by 9:00 p.m. and in bed by 10:00 p.m. Limiting screen time before heading to bed has been helpful. Also, I have realized that I can't drink caffeine after 2:00 p.m., although I swear the time keeps getting earlier and earlier!
4. **Feed my body.** I need to pay attention to added sugar, dairy, soy, and wheat, which are all known triggers that leave me feeling lackluster. I also need to be sure I'm taking my supplements and medications regularly. This example is another place where I sought help. I recognized that I wasn't feeling well after I ate sometimes. My digestion was sluggish, and I noticed my moods were being affected. I also knew that I wanted more energy without adding more caffeine just to make it through the day. So, I spoke with a women's health professional and found an approach that worked for me.
5. **Feed my senses.** Burn scented candles, buy myself flowers, soak in a warm bath with luxurious bubbles, listen to music. Fill my own cup.

6. **Move for fun.** For me, that can be dancing in the living room (80's music please!), taking a walk, or practicing yoga. I had overthought this part of my life for years, thinking that I needed to be going all-out with strenuous exercise that I didn't enjoy. Through working with my functional medicine physician, I learned that I have adrenal fatigue, so strenuous exercise was actually hurting more than helping. Make it fun, though, and I'm all in!
7. **Find the humour and laugh,** as often as possible.
8. **Feed my brain and curiosity.** Read, do puzzles, play a board game, listen to podcasts or audiobooks. Try a new food, recipe, or restaurant. Take a new route to a common destination. Change my radio station/playlist. I'm a constant learner, and curiosity is a core value that I need to honour.
9. **Open up,** both physically and metaphorically. Take deep breath breaks throughout the day, stretch, smile at the cashier and offer a warm conversation, introduce myself to a stranger. Support causes that I believe in.
10. **Be thankful.** Journal ten things every night that I'm thankful for. Some days it's not an easy exercise, but through time I've been able to notice the smallest of things, like seeing a butterfly or noticing that my husband made dinner. Being thankful keeps me focused on the positive rather than the negative.

You can see on my list that I've included the very basics of nutrition, sleep, water intake, and movement. They're so simple, but it is incredible how important they are for me to feel well; it was also amazing how often these were being ignored before I made this list!

Through working on their own list, I've seen my clients be able to step fully into their own lives with authenticity. It's permission to ask for help. It's boundary setting and learning to lovingly say "no thank you" by putting themselves first. It's also awareness around what makes them happy and how to feel fulfilled. It's the start of living your best (mid)life.

Christine Brain, Energy Healer

Think about the number of women you encounter in a day. Do any of them appear stressed? Frantic? Do you know someone dealing with anxiety or feeling depressed? What about trauma—do you know anyone whose life has been affected by a past event or events such as relationship abuse, sexual abuse, or other traumatic experience? Do you have a friend who frequently mentions headaches or migraines? Chances are you or someone you know might be challenged by a chronic or acute illness, or perhaps by being the caregiver for someone with a chronic condition.

Energy healing is the practice of directing healing energy into the body using a gentle hands-on touch technique that releases trauma, physical symptoms of pain, and emotional distress, helping women reconnect to their divine selves. The following list outlines a number of conditions or situations where energy healing offers potential benefit.

- Addiction
- Anxiety
- Depression
- Fertility
- Fears and phobias
- Grief
- Guilt
- Headaches/migraine headaches
- Insomnia

- Intrusive energies
- Limiting beliefs
- Lineage clearing
- Obsessive behaviour
- Pain management
- Past life regression
- Post Traumatic Stress Disorder
- Relationships
- Self-sabotage
- Smoking cessation
- Space clearing
- Stress
- Transitioning
- Trichotillomania (hair pulling)
- Weight management
- Worry

As I write this list, it makes what I do sound quite reactive and issue-based—and while energy healing most certainly can be a responsive or reactive practice, it can also be proactive. Energy healing sessions can deepen your state of relaxation, detoxify negative energy, and effectively raise your vibration. They can allow you to identify issues before they manifest into something unhealthy or toxic. They can help you address or avoid overwhelm.

Energy healing sessions provide excellent opportunities for self-care. They can support you by helping you nurture and navigate relationships. I have clients who specifically book sessions right before an important event, such as a job interview, or just before the holidays as a way to lessen any potential family drama, or to simply ensure a peaceful heart.

For women in midlife, energy healing provides a release for what no longer serves you and allows you to create space for whatever you wish to invite into the second half of your life. Healing is very much an individual journey, and for some women, energy healing is a successful solution for reducing stress, anxiety, challenges with sleep, and even hot flashes. Many women find energy healing to bring them vitality when they are feeling drained and joy when they are feeling down. Some describe it as a positive path to peace, self-discovery, and their "second prime."

At this point in my chapter, you are most likely either really curious, fascinated, or intrigued, or you saw the term "energy healer" and immediately became skeptical or had thoughts of "this sounds too woo-woo for me." That's okay. Trust your intuition. Get curious. Do your homework. You will know if energy healing sounds like something you might like to consider. The good news for women learning to navigate midlife is that there are many healing modalities to choose from. You are likely to find energy healing works well when integrated with other practices, including yoga, meditation, journaling, counselling, and more. You are the expert on you, and you get to design the midlife health team that can best support you on your journey.

In some communities, the practice of energy healing is regarded as "new age." The truth is, energy healing is not new. It is much older than many of the go-to health systems most of us have come to rely on today. Many native traditions speak about healing methods and insights into the layers of energy in the human body. Ancient Indian spiritual traditions and Chinese medicine practices that use energy healing date back more than 5000 years.

Energy healing encompasses a large number of well-known approaches to healing including Reiki, reflexology, and acupuncture. It also includes some lesser-known approaches such as aura and chakra balancing, crystal healing, spiritual healing, and other forms of bodywork. In my practice, I mostly provide hypnotherapy, integrative energy healing, and shamanic healing.

Shamanism is likely one of the oldest spiritual practices on earth, and its definition has certainly evolved in modern times. Essentially, it is the practice of connecting the needs of the spirit world to those of the physical world. A shamanic journey will take you into an exploration of your own inner world. Shamanism teaches you how to disconnect from the distractions of cell phones, computers, and the hectic paces of life in order to reconnect to yourself and to your community.

Integrative energy healing involves a relaxing session where you are typically awake and may participate or respond to the healer. Hypnotherapy usually involves a much deeper state of relaxation, similar to a deep meditation or even a deep sleep. The session may focus on a particular issue, such as pain, or a set of issues. A hypnotherapy session is not dramatic like what you may have seen on television; it is therapeutic, and clients often say they feel lighter, freer, and more energized as a result.

I am also an intuitive healer and clairvoyant, and I teach yoga nidra meditation and offer space clearing for homes and offices. I am able to combine my skills and customize healing sessions specifically designed for my clients. Energy healing practices can vary, and other practitioners may offer different healing modalities to choose from. It is never about one being better than the other, but rather choosing what resonates with you.

Every session is unique and designed to speak to the issues that are present in that moment in time. Energy healing works with loving grace and guides individuals to find their way back to their original intended path of good health.

My sessions begin with an intake form and a conversation about your challenges and goals. The most common length of a session is one hour, and each session is conducted in a calming environment with a massage table. Clients are fully clothed, and we recommend you wear comfortable clothing. Sometimes my hands touch your body lightly, and sometimes they pass over parts of your body I am drawn to, such as the head, chest, abdomen, and feet. Clients describe the experience as comfortable, calming, and nurturing. At the end of the session, I offer simple tips or techniques clients can practice at home. Sometimes I provide a handout or specific homework, and I always remind my clients to drink lots of water, to get plenty of rest and fresh air, and to be kind to themselves. While it might take you a few minutes to transition out of your restful state, you are able to drive and are likely to feel like you just woke from a nap.

The recommended frequency for energy healing sessions is very individual and discussed with each client. I have some clients who are working through a particular challenge who benefit from multiple sessions within a specific time frame, such as coming in once a week. Others prefer to pre-book and have their visits spread out over every few weeks or months.

I see a lot of women who are shifting. They might be shifting hormonally, making a career move, experiencing changes in their relationship or marriage, getting remarried, or becoming an empty nester or a grandmother. Even moving homes or offices can make us more energetically charged. In perimenopause, our body and our energy shifts in preparation for menopause, whether or not we are experiencing symptoms. This shift will most often affect our menstrual cycle and our mood. It might be mild and temporary, but it could be more severe and chronic.

Perimenopause is a highly sensitive time. It's a time when change begins happening in our bodies. It is also a time when we start to ask new questions of ourselves, and when we are seeking answers, receiving visions and facilitating a transformation toward the second half of our lives. Or, it could be a time in your life when things that never used to phase you suddenly become intolerable, like a family member's chewing or snoring.

I have a friend who describes midlife as this time when there is a big, bright spotlight shining down on everything we hold near and dear, and it causes us to ask and re-ask many questions. Who do I want to be? What career do I want to have? Who do I want to share my life with? What am I passionate about?

What I've learned can happen to women during this time of questioning is one of two things: they can crash and burn, or they can grow beyond their wildest expectations. And, yes, both are possible—just not at the same time! Energy healing can help you push through any blocks or challenges you may be having and help you achieve the growth you desire. Accompanied by a regular practice of mindfulness and self-care, you will realize there are no limits to your dreams.

If there is one thing I want all women to know about perimenopause (ideally before they reach perimenopause, but remember that it's never too early or too late), it's that perimenopause is a time of rebirth, but only if you allow it to be. Perimenopause has a significant purpose and role in your life, and it can be a positive one when you allow it. Perimenopause is sure to bring questions and issues to the surface for you. It will also bring answers. It's a time to clear what you no longer need, and to plant new seeds for a healthy future.

Andrea Dobbs, Cannabis Advocate

As this is being written in 2018, cannabis is enjoying a moment right now. Several US states have legalized it for recreational use, and Canada is in the process of following suit. However, while the idea of legal cannabis might be novel to some people, cannabis is not new, and the powers of the cannabis flower to treat or as relief for a variety of conditions have been documented since ancient times.

According to the Whoopi & Maya website (a medical cannabis site co-created by actress Whoopi Goldberg), there is evidence of cannabis being used to calm uterine pains dating back to the 9th century. It has been reported that Queen Victoria received a monthly dose of cannabis for menstrual discomfort throughout her adult life. In 1890 the Lancet Journal, one of the world's oldest and respected medical journals, declared cannabis to be one of the most valuable medicines for treating contractions of the uterus, commonly known as menstrual cramps.

In the early 1900s, the endocannabinoid system was discovered and named after the plant that led to its discovery. Mammals (including humans) have an endocannabinoid system, which is formally defined as a group of endogenous cannabinoid receptors located in the brain and throughout the central nervous system, consisting of neuromodulatory lipids and their receptors. In simpler terms, it is a vital system that affects just about every other bodily system, and it is involved in establishing and maintaining human health. When cannabis is consumed, chemicals found in the plant that are responsible for its effects in the mind and body, called cannabinoids, bind to these receptors and help to promote balance and self-regulation.

The Whoopi & Maya site goes on to explain how, over the years, prohibition greatly hampered cannabis research on menstrual pain and other conditions. However, the recent legal changes are renewing interest and funding for more studies on the therapeutic benefits of cannabis—particularly for women's health—including how cannabis can aid in sleep management, anxiety, digestion, memory, skin health, sexual wellness, and more.

My Story

My name is Andrea Dobbs and I am the co-founder of Village Bloomery, a dispensary I opened near Granville Island in Vancouver, British Columbia in 2015. I am a cannabis advocate. I have a strong desire to change the perceptions around cannabis and help my community, and particularly other women, achieve a healthy and balanced lifestyle. At Village Bloomery we are not only committed to the highest quality in product, we are also on a mission to ensure every customer is making informed health decisions and enjoys a positive customer experience.

In other parts of this book, you will read how perimenopause is a time of change, self-reflection, and growth. Some women leverage the perimenopause phase of life as an opportunity to tweak their lifestyle, add to or build a new health team of support, or even change careers.

I did all three.

My approach to cannabis was unconventional, to say the least. I wasn't interested in cannabis in my youth, and I felt little need to experiment with the plant in my adult life. I never really felt a need for cannabis, or any medication or that matter.

Then a bout of family stress hit and left me feeling ill-equipped to navigate the situation on my own. I was so tired, my body hurt all over, my skin was itchy, my breasts hurt, I was gaining weight, sleep was eluding me, I was dealing with acne for the first time in my life, and my sex drive had gone on an extended holiday.

And while the family stress resolved itself, as the weeks passed I discovered that I had not rebounded. Ignoring all those signals my body was giving me didn't seem like a viable strategy, so I started to research perimenopause.

On one hand, it felt good to have an understanding of the changes that were happening in my mind and in my body. On the other hand, all the new information felt quite daunting. I didn't feel as though I had adequately prepared myself for this phase of life, and the choices of "treatments" and "remedies" presented on the internet were downright overwhelming!

The first thing I did was purchase *The Hormone Cure* by Dr. Sara Gottfried. She offers some practical advice and good insight into why the body acts the way it does during this second wave of puberty.

I found great success with cutting out coffee, adding adrenal supplementation, and adding kelp to my diet to support my thyroid. I also reduced my sugar intake dramatically, added a vitamin B complex supplement, and really started to pay attention to and intentionally slow down my busy lifestyle. I did yoga, upped my walking, started hiking, and rode my bike more often. Dr. Gottfried's protocol recommends what she refers to as a pyramid approach, with lifestyle tweaks (paying attention to how we eat, move, sleep and manage stress) as the essential bottom layer of the pyramid. The next layer includes adding high quality vitamins and supplements that may be missing from your diet, and the top layer—which is optional—is exploring any other external support, method, or modality that will address your specific needs. This could include everything from counselling to hormone therapy.

Within a matter of a few weeks, it felt as though a film was lifting from my eyes. My world was starting to look a little brighter and I had more energy, but my body still didn't feel quite like my own so I continued to look for options.

I have always been interested in plant-based medicine, especially when it comes to my own personal health. I have consulted with more alternative health practitioners (naturopath/homeopathic/acupuncturist/chiropractic) than I have conventional ones. Therefore, my research followed that route as well.

While surfing the Internet one day, I stumbled across an article that spoke of THC's relationship with progesterone and the ways cannabis can affect the menstrual cycle, and it piqued my interest.

After reading the article, I decided that THC was for me. Although I had tried smoking a few times in my adult life, I had never enjoyed the experience or the outcome so I was not a casual consumer. However, this new information set me on a mission. I walked into a local cannabis shop and began to share my story with the young male attendant, whose face slowly lost its colour and whose eyes were cast down to the counter as I repeated my questions about periods, PMS, and perimenoapuse.

He slid me a chocolate and said, "A lot of women buy these for PMS. It might work."

I gave it a shot. The chocolate tasted a bit dirty but generally it was tolerable. I waited and waited for something to happen, and then assumed that I would need to smoke in order to feel the effect I was seeking.

My daughters and I were on our way to shop for grad shoes when a wave of "WOW" hit me. Suddenly, I had to slump down onto the sofa, and I laid there for what must have been hours, drooling. The girls were not impressed. Neither was I.

Eventually the "WOW" became a "Hmmm..." and I thought to myself, "This doesn't feel so bad…in fact, it feels pretty good."

The young fellow in the cannabis shop was not entirely wrong with his recommendation, but his information around dosage and application were lacking.

This experience marked the beginning of my cannabis journey. Eventually, I leveraged my cannabis education to switch careers and open my own shop.

What You Should Know about Cannabis

Are you curious about cannabis? No doubt you've been familiar with the plant for years—53% of Canadian adults have some personal consumption experience with cannabis [BDS Analytics]. You've probably heard all the nicknames, stereotypes, and euphemisms too. Pot. Weed. Grass. Mary Jane. Let's get clear on definitions, discuss modalities and then share options for experimenting and/or introducing cannabis into your midlife health plan.

While the scientists debate these definitions, its generally accepted that there are three types of cannabis plants: indica, sativa, and ruderalis. We'll stick to the two main types, indica and sativa.

Indica plants are typically relaxing and calming. They can be used for sedation, relieving pain, and reducing stress relievers. In contrast, sativa plants are typically uplifting, creative, euphoric, happy, and activating.

The term "strain" is used to describe different cannabis plants. Pure plants are called landrace strains, while plants that have been crossbred are called hybrid strains. There are over 1,000 strains, and at any given time, we have twenty to thirty strains in our store.

Phenotypes are like children: every cannabis seed is a different phenotype of the strain. An experienced grower will sprout several seeds, take clippings from them each, and grow those "clones" to flowering plants. These plants are then tested, and the grower picks the one (or more) he likes the best. This is now his phenotype of the strain. Often, the strain that smells the best to you will give you the best benefits.

There are two main active ingredients, or cannabinoids, that are found in cannabis. **Tetrahydrocannabinol (THC)** is the main psychoactive element in the plant and is the one that is most commonly known. It has many uses, including as an analgesic (pain reliever), anti-inflammatory, anti-oxidant, neuroprotective/neuroregenerative, antiemetic (anti-nausea), sleep-aid, appetite stimulant, and more.

Cannabidiol (CBD) is the second most plentiful cannabinoid and is actually an anti-psychotic, reducing the euphoric effects of THC while making the benefits last longer. CBD is non-intoxicating and has many properties, including anticonvulsive/antispasmodic, anti-inflammatory, neuroprotective/neuroregenerative, anti-depressant, muscle relaxant, sedative, anti-anxiety, and relieving some forms of high blood pressure.

Modalities and Delivery Methods

There are a few common ways that cannabis is consumed. **Inhalation** is the most immediate way to deliver the benefits of cannabis. For this reason, it can be effective in treating asthma, nausea, pain, migraine headaches, and anxiety attacks. It takes from five to fifteen minutes to fully feel an inhaled dose, and the effects may last an hour or two. Inhaling is the most common method of reaching a euphoric ("high") effect.

Ingestion is common if you are looking for longer-term effects. It can also be one of the more challenging ways to consume as timing and dosage are key. It can take up to two hours to fully feel the benefits of an edible dose, and the effect can last for several hours. If the goal is staying asleep, ingestion may be the preferred mode of delivery.

Absorbing cannabis topicals can be effective in delivering pain management as well as treating skin conditions such as rosacea, eczema, and psoriasis. New users often prefer the ease of trying topicals without having to inhale or ingest the dose.

Oral dosing by either consuming cannabis sublingually (under the tongue) or buccally (through the cheeks) is a quick way to deliver the benefits. Relief can often be felt from within a few seconds up to twenty minutes and may last for two to three hours depending on your dose. This method is most often preferred by those who need quick effects but don't enjoy inhaling, or who need a more discrete method. Sprays are convenient and effective for reducing stress and anxiety. Tinctures (alcohol infused with cannabis extract) are common for inducing sleep and are also effective and convenient.

Inserting cannabis (as a suppository vaginally or rectally) can be a highly effective delivery method with a quick response time and a fraction of the intoxication of an equivalent edible dose. Inserts are considered useful for managing painful menstruation, irritable bowel conditions, or as part of cancer therapy.

Andrea's Own Midlife Health Protocol

Women often come into Village Bloomery with an air of purpose. "I want to sleep!" is a common greeting. While we would love to say we have their magic solution, that would be remiss. The truth is there is magic to be experienced, but a one-size-fits-all sleep remedy does not exist.

I have learned through experience that women are hungry for information, and they are eager to participate in managing their own health and be proactive in achieving wellness—in midlife and beyond! They are often challenged by the fact that fifteen minutes in their doctor's office did not leave them feeling empowered to do so. I want to share my experience of navigating perimenopause in an effort to empower and inspire others.

For my skin: I had very itchy skin, especially on my shins. To manage this, I regularly moisturize with either a THC-infused massage oil or coconut oil, depending if I want to smell pretty or if smelling slightly earthy and tropical is okay. This moisturizing has helped immensely. In fact, I've not had itchy skin in over two years. I've also not had an acne break out in that time frame as well, which is a nice benefit.

For my aches and pains: I've never been diagnosed with any type of chronic pain, but pain manages to sneak up on me from time to time. It shows up in my forearms, in my hands and feet, and in my knees and shoulders. It is not constant, and it isn't debilitating, but it is bothersome. The topical application of oil helps in the short-term, but I find better relief in micro-dosing CBD and THC. I take 7.5 mg of THC and CBD every morning, and I often take another 5 mg between 4:00–6:00 p.m. Please note: always follow the dosage recommendations of an experienced professional. I worked my way up to this dose slowly over a period of time. I've also found that I have to avoid eating nightshades (potatoes, tomatoes, eggplant, peppers) as I've realized they definitely impact my pain, so whenever I do, my regular THC and CBD dose needs to be increased too.

Though there are many options for low-dose products, I generally choose the infused coconut oil in the morning with my blender latte, and a 1:1 capsule in the evening. I rotate a group of other products into my routine when needed, including 5mg THC capsules, the CBD tincture, the 1:1 and 4:1 tincture, and the super micro-dose Cannatonic tincture.

I also use topical ointments that are either a full THC, a 1:1 or full CBD profile. I rotate through these based on where I have pain, how strong I need it to be, and whether or not the smell matters to me. When approaching my period, I use the same infused massage oil I use for my itchy skin for my sore breasts.

For sleep: I found that my sleep improved a ton when I eliminated coffee, and it has become even better since I've been able to wean myself down to under three grams of added sugar a day. I eat fruit, honey, and maple syrup, but I limit refined sugars and do not consume any artificial sweeteners.

On the odd night that I have way too much on my mind, I will take an Indica tincture. My personal favourite is Cronica Farms Pink K Tincture. I don't have a reason for why it's my personal favourite, other than that I like the packaging and it works for me! This alcohol-based tincture activates quickly and allows my mind to calm down, guiding me to an easy sleep. An infused tincture is always good for me as well, though I tend to save them for when I'm in need some extra tender loving care.

For my libido: My libido came back almost in sync with my improved sleep patterns and when my body no longer itched or hurt. Generally I was "good to go," but there was lots of media chatter about Sutra-infused lubricants and I was curious. They are good. They are really, really good!

If you are working to find your libido, these lubricants are a great place to start looking. The oil is placed on the clitoris and takes about fifteen minutes to make a "connection." The connection is equivalent to a thought or an idea. Then, blood flow increases and there is a moment where the pleasure centres awaken. That's when I suggest masturbating or engaging with your partner—you are almost guaranteed to awaken zones that have been under wraps for a while! This might not be the only step you need to restore your libido, but I would definitely recommend giving it a try.

If you experience pain with penetration, lack of lubrication, and/or thinning and inflammation of the vaginal walls, a vaginal suppository about one hour before intimacy can relax the muscles, reduce swelling, ease any pain, and encourage lubrication. By inserting THC into the vagina daily, you will likely find relief from vaginal atrophy as well.

For my energy levels: I do generally have much more energy than before I started paying attention to my health, but there are still days where I feel a little low. I might not feel like getting out of bed, and I don't want to go to yoga or jump on the elliptical machine. That is typically when I will take my Sativa tincture. I usually take about 7.5 mg of this tincture when I need that extra boost, and within seconds I'm feeling revitalized. It's my favourite replacement for coffee.

For fun: many women in my life, and in midlife, turn to wine for fun and self-medication. I am all about having fun. Since I am off sugar, I am also off conventional alcoholic beverages. This can leave me feeling excluded at times, so when it comes to attending social functions, I choose the Sativa tincture if I want that "champagne" feeling and an Indica tincture if I'm looking for a red wine vibe. I love the vapour pens that are out in the marketplace because they are often pretty and discreet, that said we have to wait a while for those to come back as they are not available in the legal marketplace just yet.

After reading this, I'm hopeful that you'll feel empowered to explore your own health in a practical and experimental way. This is my perspective, and like with any medicine, cannabis requires some trial and experimentation. Do discuss your questions with experts. The amount of research and educational resources is only going to continue to increase. It's important to allow yourself the time to find your holy grail.

Dr. Anna Garrett, Hormone Balance Expert

I am a certified coach, a doctor of pharmacy, and hormone balance expert, and I am passionate about working with women who want to make their health a priority. I'm also navigating my own midlife journey. I see clients one-on-one, both in person and online, to help them navigate their perimenopause-to-menopause journey. They are often challenged by poor sleep, fatigue, anxiety, weight gain, and mood swings—all common perimenopause experiences. Together, we create a custom solution that fits with their lifestyle, allows them to achieve the results they are looking for, and gets their mojo back on track!

Women will often arrive at our appointments saying one of two things: "Do I need to have my hormone levels tested?" Or, "I asked my doctor if I could have my hormone levels tested and he said no."

There is so much confusing and conflicting information online and in the medical community when it comes to navigating perimenopause and menopause. To help combat this, I am going to share my knowledge of the various available options for hormone testing, what you can expect from each one, some of the pros and cons, and even what you might expect to learn from hormone testing, depending on which care provider you see. I hope that you can use this information to be your own best health advocate and empower yourself to be able to talk to your doctor about hormones and hormone testing with confidence.

What I am NOT going to tell you is which tests you need or don't need, as that is a decision to be made between you and your physician/health care professional.

Before I do that, I want to describe two scenarios to help you understand the different approaches people or even health care professionals might take in regards to hormones.

The first scenario is that of a road trip. I'm sure you can picture it: suitcases packed, convertible top down, sunglasses on, your BFF riding shotgun beside you. The question is: do you need a map?

For some women, the answer might be no. They aren't on a specific time line, they don't have a specific destination in mind, and they will pull over to the side of the road when they need to figure out their direction. Some things might go well, some things might not, and they are kind of half-prepared for either. Basically, they have decided to wing the entire trip without a road map.

For other women, this isn't the type of journey they need at this time in their lives. They do have a specific time line and a specific set of goals. They want a plan mapped out for them that will show them where they started and what they experienced along the route. When they arrive at their destination, they will be able to look back and appreciate how far they've come.

When it comes to hormone conversations, testing is one tool that a health care professional has in their toolkit. Testing is intended to be used in combination with conversations with the patient about other health conditions and the symptoms that are the most concerning. Health care professionals like to use testing to validate a certain set of assumptions ("Her symptoms make me think she is experiencing estrogen dominance"), or question/rule out other possibilities ("I'm not sure if her depressed feelings and inability to concentrate are related to fluctuations in progesterone or a thyroid condition"). Testing can also be beneficial in determining a baseline for a woman so she knows what "normal" looks like for her. If she is going to introduce a new protocol, such as supplementation and/or hormone therapy, she and her health care professional will be able to refer back to her baseline test to monitor and track results. Test results act like the beginning of your trip planning; they are directional; a road map if you will.

My second analogy is related to travel as well. We can all imagine that feeling of driving in your car and glancing down at the dashboard, only to realize your CHECK ENGINE light is on. It can be alarming as thoughts cross in and out of your mind, ranging from "Oh God, it's something serious." to "I'm sure it's nothing." You drive straight to your local mechanic's shop to explain to him that your engine light has just come on and it's a concern for you. He has two options. He can put some duct tape over the light, or he can lift the hood and investigate what triggered the light and what the root cause might be. Both options get rid of the light on your dash. Which will you prefer?

When a woman is experiencing hormone fluctuations in perimenopause, it can lead to symptoms that might be mildly noticeable or moderately inconvenient. For approximately 20% of women, these symptoms can become severe and disruptive to her quality of life. Symptoms are your body's way of alerting you that something is off and requires your attention, and that something may need a gentle tweak or a course correction. Rather than masking the symptom with a band-aid or duct tape, "looking under the hood" for the root cause and treating whatever is causing the symptom is likely to result in a better health outcome. Hormone testing helps physicians confirm their hypothesis and uncover any underlying root causes.

I speak with so many women who are frustrated when their doctors don't see the value in testing hormone levels. It's a common story, and it's important for women to understand the following:

- Testing for menopause is unnecessary. Rarely do you need a test to determine if you've reached menopause. The answer to whether you've reached menopause lies in whether or not it has been twelve months since your final menstrual period.

Exceptions would be for a woman who has had a partial hysterectomy, or for a woman who is making a new decision about birth control and needs confirmation.

- Testing is not always a prerequisite for treatment. Every woman is different, and so is every health care professional. Some doctors feel confident prescribing hormone therapy or a new health protocol to certain patients who present with classic symptoms. For example, if a woman's chief complaint is vaginal dryness, she doesn't need a hormone test to confirm that she needs treatment!
- Hormone testing is a snapshot in time. Our hormones—especially in perimenopause—are fluctuating all the time. They vary from month-to-month, week-to-week, day-to-day and even hour-to-hour. You could test in the morning and again at night and produce different results. For this reason, hormone testing is considered a guide or a support rather than the definitive be-all answer to your concerns. A trained clinician will look at your lab results and look for patterns, analyze the magnitude of any hormone imbalances, and also look to see if there are any alarm bells that may not have come up while taking the patient history.

It is also important to be aware that in some cases, there may be a cost involved in receiving hormone testing. In the US, the cost for testing hormones will vary depending on your insurance coverage. In Canada, there are tests, such as blood tests, that your family physician can order that will be covered under your medical services plan. If you are working with a naturopath or other health care professional, you will likely have to pay for the hormone testing out of pocket. I have started to hear many success stories of integrated health teams working together on solutions that are best for the patient. For example, your naturopath may request certain tests, and it's possible that you can ask your family doctor to order those tests without the out-of-pocket expense. I do love the concept of a collaborative approach to women's health and we are seeing more and more examples, which is promising.

As I mentioned, testing hormone levels is only one tool that your health professional has to help guide and recommend the best protocol for you and your particular situation. Your doctor might not be trained in hormone balance and may be hesitant due to a lack of experience or confidence that he/she will know what to do with the results. If you've determined that hormone testing might be beneficial for you and you have been met with some resistance, there are good examples of approaches you can take to the conversation on page 38 of this book.

There are three main types of tests: saliva, blood and urine or dried urine. **Saliva testing** identifies free hormone levels, is non-invasive, is great for tests that require multiple collections, and is the preferred method of many naturopaths and alternative health care providers. Collection can be done at home with minimal instructions, no freezing or refrigeration is required, and samples are stable at room temperature for thirty days. Saliva testing is effective for monitoring hormone therapy that is administered orally, vaginally, or via pellets, as well as for determining cortisol levels for adrenal stress assessment. It is not effective for women who have dry mouth syndrome.

Blood tests are commonly requisitioned by family doctors and are considered the ideal method for measuring molecular structures too large to capture in saliva, such as blood lipids, vitamin D and thyroid hormones. Blood testing is a broadly accepted method for measuring hormone levels but is not effective for monitoring topical or vaginal hormone therapy.

Dried urine testing is my preferred testing method. It provides the best way to measure hormone by-products and provides the only gauge for measuring how the body is metabolizing its hormones. Dried urine testing allows for discreet, at-home collection and only requires four to five samples, which eliminates the disadvantages of the hourly urine collections that were previously necessary for the older twenty-four-hour urine testing. Dried urine testing is suitable for measuring hormone levels, assessing cortisol production at four time points for stress assessment, and measuring melatonin production. It is not suitable for the ongoing monitoring of topical or vaginal hormone therapy.

Shirley often asks her network of women's health professionals, "What do you want women to know about perimenopause?" I believe it's important for all women to have this information on hormone testing so they can have more informed, productive, and engaged conversations with their health team. Are you expected to know what tests to order, or what method of collection would be best or what the numbers mean on your lab results? Absolutely not. That's a job for someone like me. Are you expected to be the captain of your own midlife team? One hundred percent! In order to be proactive and an advocate for your own health, you do need to understand the context of the conversation and what your options are.

Know this: there is no hormone test that can tell you or your doctor what treatment protocol or dosage is right for you. Hormone balance is very individual, and tests, as we've discussed, are merely a guide. I always recommend you work with an experienced professional who can not only request and interpret your test results, but who can also recommend nutritional and lifestyle options, with or without the inclusion of hormone therapy.

Jennifer Howker, Registered Dietitian

You are unique. How *your* body digests, absorbs, and uses food is different from anyone else. Unfortunately, in a world where false or questionable claims about nutrition are easily accessible and ubiquitous, figuring out what is good or relevant can be difficult and confusing. A registered dietitian (RD) or professional dietitian (PD) can help you to avoid the problems that can result from acting on dietary misinformation and nutritional myths, and to determine the best dietary approach for *your* body with *your* goals and lifestyle in mind.

A dietitian analyzes your nutrient needs during different life stages and makes recommendations to prevent or manage disease and minimize symptoms if necessary. During the perimenopause and menopause stages, for example, the accompanying hormonal fluctuations cause changes in our bodies, including increased weight, loss of bone density, increased risk for heart disease, increased risk for breast cancer, and symptoms ranging from hot flashes and insomnia to forgetfulness.

A dietitian employs his or her expertise to make recommendations that are realistic and consistent with your personal health and life goals. For example, if you are approaching menopause, want to train for an upcoming 10k run, have chosen not to use hormone replacement therapy (HRT), and have a strong family history of breast cancer, your nutrition plan will be different than if your main goal is to decrease the severity and frequency of hot flashes and mood swings and manage your Type 2 diabetes. There isn't one nutrition plan that is suitable or ideal for everyone. For this reason, it is worth the effort to find a qualified nutrition expert and make him or her an integral part of your health care team.

Finding a Dietitian

Many people claim to be nutrition experts, but when you are looking for one with the qualifications to look after your nutritional health needs, you should know the titles "dietitian," "registered dietitian," and "professional dietitian" are protected by law across Canada (just like "physician," "nurse," and "pharmacist"). This means they may only be used by qualified practitioners who have met rigorous educational qualifications. Specifically, dietitians must have a Bachelor of Science degree in Human Nutrition and complete an internship (and/or master's degree) that has been approved by their provincial regulatory body. Dietitians must also meet and maintain provincial registration requirements in addition to educational accreditation, including proof of continued competency in the field of human nutrition.

Dietitians who have met the national standards for education and training and who are members of their provincial regulatory bodies can use one of the following designations: RD, RDN, PDt, or RDt (or the French equivalent, DtP). There are other professionals who may have varying degrees of nutrition expertise, but enlisting the help of a dietitian is one way you can guarantee that you have someone on your medical team with a solid understanding of human nutrition, including digestion, absorption, and metabolism through the life cycle and surrounding various chronic health conditions.

Many health authorities offer outpatient dietitian counselling, but the wait is often lengthy and follow-up appointments may be difficult to book. Thus, you may need to do your own search for a dietitian, in which case you can use the Dietitians of Canada website to look for private practice dietitians in your area. You can also use the Menopause Chicks "Find an Expert" directory or access the dietetics governing body in your province or area. If you have specific dietary issues resulting from certain medical conditions (for example, celiac disease), you may wish to seek out an RD with expertise in that area. Many health insurance plans cover RD visits.

A dietitian will use your medical history, a physical examination, your diet history, and recent blood work to rule out possible or likely nutrition deficiencies. He or she will also be able to identify which of your medications may affect your body's ability to absorb, store, or use different nutrients.

Preparing for Your First Visit

Prior to your first visit with an RD, it's a good idea to prepare by gathering some key information if you can; otherwise, a large portion of your initial visit may need to be spent gathering the information the RD needs in order to help you. If possible, it's helpful to provide the RD with the following information at or prior to your initial visit.

Seven-day food diary

Make a list of all the food you consume over a seven-day period. This record should include:

- The time of day (or night) the food was consumed. Don't forget snacks and beverages!
- What kind of food was consumed.
- What is my portion size. (Try to be as accurate as you can and measure or weigh portions if possible.)

It is also important to advise the dietitian of any food allergies, intolerances, or foods you may avoid for cultural, ethical, or any other reasons.

The more detailed you can be, the better. For example, for a cup of coffee, you might write, "Eight ounces of coffee with one tablespoon of cream and one teaspoon of sugar." It is also helpful to record the cooking method—whether your meal is grilled, roasted, or fried can significantly affect its nutrient profile. Please be as honest as possible and include any alcohol you consume as this can have a significant effect on your caloric intake and micronutrient status.

There is no need for you to make any dietary changes at this point. The seven-day food record is just meant to capture your typical intake and identify any habits or patterns.

Recent blood test results

If possible, bring a copy of your latest blood work (ideally drawn within the past month). Also, if you have any recent test results for a suspected nutrient deficiency, it's very useful to include those as well. You may need to ask your doctor or naturopathic practitioner to refer you for such tests. For example, if you have noticed you are more tired than usual and your skin appears pale, or if your basic blood work is suggestive of an iron deficiency (low hemoglobin), you can ask your doctor to add "iron studies" to your basic blood work to help confirm or rule out iron deficiency anemia.

Blood work can reveal a lot about your nutrition and health status and helps take away some of the guess work that would otherwise be required. It can also provide a starting point for your physician or RD to identify specific health patterns (baseline levels, highs, lows) over time, or through life stages such as perimenopause and menopause.

List of current medications and supplements

Make a list of any medications or supplements you are taking. Include vitamin and mineral supplements, probiotics, and any herbal supplements or meal replacements you may take. Many medications and herbal supplements can affect nutrient absorption or availability in the body. Conversely, many nutrients and nutrition supplements can affect the ability of a medication to do its intended job.

Personal medical history

Describe any chronic illnesses you may have, including any sensitivities or recurring issues with your GI tract—for example, constipation or diarrhea, acid reflux, and excessive gas or bloating. These can all provide valuable clues as to what is going on in your digestive tract in terms of the digestion and absorption of nutrients. Include any other ongoing health issues you can think of, including skin conditions, allergies or sensitivities, numbness or tingling, heavy bleeding during menstruation (menorrhagia), or even changes in mood or cognitive function.

Family medical history

Report all significant family history for major health concerns, including mental illness, autoimmune conditions, or any other chronic illness. Any family history of heart disease, breast cancer, or osteoporosis is particularly important, as the hormonal changes experienced by menopausal or perimenopausal women (such as declining estrogen levels) tend to increase the health risks associated with these conditions.

Physical assessment

Your RD will likely do a physical assessment to rule out any obvious nutrient deficiencies that have resulted in (usually subtle) physical abnormalities. In addition to the history you provide, the state of your hair, skin, nails, and mouth can all provide valuable information regarding your current nutrition status.

Case Study: Michelle

There are several areas in which a menopausal or perimenopausal woman's health and quality of life are significantly impacted by her nutritional status. A dietitian will assist by assessing your diet, symptoms, lifestyle, and risk factors. Using this information, the RD will identify your potential nutrition issues and develop realistic nutrition strategies to help manage your symptoms and achieve your personal health goals.

To help illustrate the process of nutrition assessment and nutrition plan development, let's examine the case of Michelle.

Michelle is a forty-eight-year-old mother who works from home full time. She lives with her husband and two kids (age thirteen and fifteen). Her work day starts very early because many of her clients are in Eastern Canada, where the time zones are three or four hours ahead of where she lives on B.C.'s coast. Her kids are very active in sports, which means Michelle drives them to various practices and games most evenings and weekends, leaving limited time for meal preparation and sit-down meals.

She has trouble falling asleep, and night sweats are contributing to her poor quality of sleep. She is experiencing headaches and mood swings that are concerning to her and her family. She is frustrated by her "foggy brain" and feels generally stressed and emotional. She has gained weight steadily over the past five years and is finding it increasingly difficult to lose. She walks daily and jogs two times per week for about thirty minutes each time. Her body mass index (BMI) is twenty-nine, which is defined as being overweight. She is still menstruating most months, and her menstrual flow is increasing in heaviness as she approaches menopause.

Her family history is negative for breast cancer and osteoporosis. However, Michelle's father passed away from heart disease.

Michelle has a strong aversion to swallowing pills but has been taking 40 mg of esomeprazole (an acid-reducing medication, commonly sold under the brand name Nexium) once a day for the past two years to deal with GERD (gastroesophageal reflux disease or acid reflux). Other than this, she is not currently on any medications, vitamin/mineral supplements, probiotics, or herbal remedies. She would like to keep it this way and is motivated to meet her nutrition needs through food intake.

Michelle's typical daily nutritional intake

5:00 a.m.: Gets up, drinks a six-ounce glass of water, walks for thirty minutes.

5:30 a.m.: Drinks two eight-ounce cups of coffee, each with two tablespoons of 18% cream and no sugar.

7:00 a.m.: Eats three quarters of a cup of supermarket "probiotic" yogurt with thirty grams of granola and a half cup of frozen berries, along with one cup of coffee with cream (as above).

9:00 a.m.: Eats one medium banana and drinks a six-ounce cup of coffee with two tablespoons 18% cream.

12:30 p.m.: Eats a grilled cheese or ham sandwich or a whole wheat bun with butter, along with a salad consisting of two cups of mixed greens (lettuce and spinach) with half a cup of chopped chicken, one third of a cup of cucumber, half an ounce of feta cheese, and two tablespoons of dressing. Drinks an eight-ounce cup of water or tea.

2:00 p.m.: Eats ten to twelve crackers or one cup tortilla chips with one to two ounces of cheese, one to two ounces of chocolate, and drinks one cup of black tea with no cream or sugar.

4:00-5:00 p.m.: Michelle makes dinner and typically snacks while doing so. By completing her diet history, she realized she was consuming a significant amount of calories (300-500) at this time without adding much nutritive value. Her snacks of choice typically included high salt, high fat foods like potato chips, cheezies, or cookies.

Michelle takes her stomach acid reducing medication just before dinner to relieve the acid reflux she experiences later in the evening.

5:00-6:00 p.m.: Michelle and family eat dinner, which is typically very "kid friendly"—high in fat, salt, and carbohydrates (macaroni and cheese, frozen pizza, meatloaf with potatoes and vegetables like carrots or cucumber slices, tacos, or grilled cheese sandwiches).

7:00 p.m.: Eats three cups of microwave popcorn and drinks one to two glasses of white wine.

9:00 p.m.: Eats three quarters of a cup of ice cream.

Comparison to the *Canada's Food Guide* recommendations

The rationale behind the *Canada's Food Guide* (CFG) recommendations is ensuring that your diet provides the estimated daily amounts of macronutrients (fat, carbohydrates [including fiber] and protein) and micronutrients (vitamins, minerals, trace elements, antioxidants, and phytonutrients) required to support good health. Although micronutrients are only required in tiny (micro) amounts, they are vital in preventing serious health problems.

A comparison of how Michelle's diet measures up against CFG gives us some more clues as to which nutrients her diet may be lacking.

Food Group	Canada's Food Guide # of servings recommended per day (for women ages 19-50)	Michelle's current typical intake	Macronutrients suspected to be lacking in Michelle's diet	Micronutrients suspected to be lacking in Michelle's diet
Fruits and vegetables	7-8	5 (mostly fruit)	Fiber	Phytochemicals, antioxidants
Grain products	6-7	4-8 (mostly white, processed)	Fiber, omega 3 fats	Several B vitamins, iron, magnesium
Milk and alternatives	2 (including 2 cups of milk or milk substitute)	2 (no milk)	Protein	Calcium, vitamins D and B12
Meat and alternatives	2	1-2	Protein, omega 3 fat	B12, iron, isoflavones (soy)

Looking at Michelle's diet history, it is clear there are some food groups (and therefore nutrients) that she isn't getting enough of. We can see that she needs to increase her intake of vegetables, whole grains, fiber, protein, and omega-3 fats. While she is getting two servings of milk alternatives, neither of these servings include milk or a fortified soy beverage to ensure adequate vitamin D intake. We can also determine that Michelle is not getting enough calcium, magnesium, or iron from her diet most days.

Her caffeine, saturated fat, and salt (sodium) intakes are excessive. Combined, these foods will contribute to a number of Michelle's perimenopausal symptoms including decreased bone density, hot flashes, irritability, poor sleep, and increased risk of heart disease

Blood work provides more clues to what is going on with Michelle.

The following table provides a summary of Michelle's recent results ordered by her family physician.

Test	Michelle's results	What it measures
Red blood cell (RBC) count	**low**	How many red blood cells present in a given volume of blood
Hemoglobin	**low**	The amount of hemoglobin (an iron-rich molecule that carries oxygen to the tissues) in a given volume of blood
Serum iron	**normal**	Iron in blood
LDL cholesterol	**high**	Serum levels of low-density (harmful) lipoprotein
HDL cholesterol	**low**	Serum levels of high-density (beneficial) lipoprotein
Non-HDL cholesterol	**high**	All cholesterol other than HDL
Triglycerides (TG)	**high**	Serum levels of sugar/cholesterol molecule

It is important to note that the esomeprazole Michelle takes for acid reflux has some significant nutrition implications. Because esomeprazole is an acid reducer, it affects the body's ability to absorb B12, which needs to be activated by acid in the stomach prior to absorption in the small intestine. Studies have shown that long-term (more than one year) use of this type of medication can also cause low magnesium and calcium levels and increase the risk for bone fractures.

Putting it all together

As Michelle's dietitian, I analyzed her nutritional intake, blood work, medical history, lifestyle, and personal health goals and preferences, and decided that we need to focus on the following areas.

Iron:

Michelle's blood work indicates that she has a low RBC and low hemoglobin—results consistent with possible iron deficiency anemia. Iron is important, not only as a component of hemoglobin (the molecule that carries oxygen around in our blood), but also as a component in certain neurotransmitters in the brain that are known to affect your ability to concentrate, learn, and regulate mood. An iron deficiency could certainly explain some of Michelle's symptoms, but iron supplements aren't always well tolerated so I don't like to recommend them without careful consideration of the client's needs—especially when, like Michelle, she is averse to the idea of taking supplements.

Because Michelle's food diary and blood work are both indicative of a possible iron deficiency—and because Michelle was experiencing increasing fatigue, heavy menstrual flow (increased iron losses), and low mood—it would be worthwhile to have her ferritin checked. Ferritin is the storage form of iron in the body and can be depleted significantly before a low serum iron is detectable in basic blood work.

Vitamin B12:

Interpreting blood work is more challenging when more than one type of anemia or illness is present. A deficiency in B12 is called pernicious anemia and can be difficult to detect using basic blood work when there is also iron deficiency anemia present. We can use the diet history, medical history, and family history to help determine the likelihood of a deficiency and then request a serum B12 level if warranted. In Michelle's case, her dietary B12 intake is on the low side and her medication affects her ability to absorb B12. In addition to this, we know that the ability to absorb B12 decreases with age.

Many of Michelle's symptoms can be explained, at least in part, by a B12 deficiency, including headaches, difficulty falling asleep (B12 is known to influence melatonin release and metabolism), cognitive changes, and mood swings.

Magnesium:

Magnesium is essential in regulating many diverse biochemical reactions in the body, including protein synthesis, muscle and nerve function, blood glucose control, and blood pressure regulation. It contributes to the structural development of our bones and is required for the synthesis of DNA.

I suspect Michelle's magnesium status to be low, despite the fact that there is no accurate way to confirm this with a blood test. Serum magnesium doesn't tell us much about the body's magnesium status. In fact, serum magnesium can be within a normal range while the rest of the body is working at a magnesium deficit. The symptoms of low magnesium—fatigue, weakness, muscle cramps—are non-specific, which contributes to the difficulty of diagnosing a deficiency.

What we *do* know is that Michelle's diet is likely low in magnesium, and that long-term use of esomeprazole is known to cause low magnesium levels.

Heart disease:

Michelle's low-density lipoprotein (LDL—the "bad" cholesterol) is elevated and her high-density lipoprotein (HDL—"good" cholesterol) is low. These risk factors are concerning, given her positive family history for heart disease, her additional risk factor of having a body mass index (BMI) over twenty-five, and the fact that her estrogen levels are now starting to drop.

Michelle's diet history shows there is certainly room for improvement in terms of dietary changes that could help prevent heart disease. Limiting saturated fat (typically animal fat) and trans fat intake, increasing omega-3 fat intake, and increasing vegetables and fibre will all have a protective effect on her heart.

Osteoporosis:

Although Michelle hasn't done a bone mass density test and she doesn't have a family history of osteoporosis, there are several risk factors for this condition that are of concern.

Estrogen is important in the maintenance of bone density and strength, so it makes sense that through perimenopause, when our estrogen levels start fluctuating, bone loss increases along with the risk of fractures. In addition, Michelle's dietary calcium, vitamin D, and magnesium intake are inadequate; also, esomeprazole can negatively affect calcium and magnesium absorption and therefore result in decreasing bone density.

Recommendations for Michelle

Have bone density tested:

Michelle should have her bone density tested to provide a baseline measurement for future reference. This will help Michelle and her health team determine how her bone density is changing over time and can also help determine the effectiveness of any future treatment for osteoporosis.

Increase daily exercise:

I recommend that Michelle start a regimen of exercise, including weight-bearing exercise, not only to help with weight loss but also to improve her bone density, stamina, sleep, and mood. A good personal trainer would be able to help develop a program suitable for a perimenopausal woman like Michelle.

Re-evaluate the need for esomeprazole:

Medications such as acid reducers are prescribed by the GP to deal with a symptom or health issue that is relevant at the time, but sometimes they are continued well beyond the point at which they are no longer required or a much lower dose would suffice. Michelle is now making dietary changes that should decrease her symptoms of acid reflux.

If she does still experience reflux, there are other medications with fewer nutrient interactions that could be considered. A pharmacist is a great resource for this kind of information.

Have ferritin and serum B12 tested:

Having Michelle's ferritin and serum B12 levels tested will let us know whether she suffers from iron deficiency anemia, pernicious anemia or both.

Nutrition plan:

Keeping in mind that Michelle is not keen on taking supplements, I would make the following nutrition recommendations:

1. **Start tracking food intake:** Use an online tool or app such as MyFitnessPal or Lose It! to track food intake. This is a very good way to increase your attentiveness to food and nutrition and is a powerful tool for weight loss.
2. **Incorporate soy foods:** Adding soy foods to her daily diet should help Michelle with her hot flashes, decrease her risk of heart disease, and help minimize the effect of menopause on her bone density. Edamame, soy beverages, tofu, and soy protein powder are all good choices.
3. **Increase intake of omega-3 fats:** Michelle should enjoy fatty fish two to three times per week and use ground flax seeds

and/or flax seed oil daily. This will provide the cardio-protective omega-3 fats that will help lower her risk of heart disease. Omega-3 fats can also help with mood swings and depressive symptoms.

4. **Increase fiber intake:** Michelle should increase her intake of dietary fiber by switching to whole-grain breads, cereals, rice, and pasta. Fiber is known to help decrease cholesterol levels and will also help Michelle feel fuller after a meal, thus decreasing the likelihood of overeating and contributing to weight loss.
5. **Decrease saturated fat intake:** Reducing her intake of saturated fats will help Michelle lower her cholesterol levels and assist with her weight loss efforts. One way for Michelle to do this is to switch from 18% cream to 6% cream in her coffee. She could also choose lower fat cheese and modify some of her recipes by substituting low-saturated-fat ingredients where necessary.
6. **Increase intake of vegetables:** Eating more vegetables will help increase Michelle's dietary fiber and provide an impressive amount and variety of micronutrients in the form of vitamins, antioxidants, and minerals.
7. **Increase magnesium intake:** Michelle should replace the empty calories of her current snack food choices with high-magnesium foods such as nuts, spinach, whole grain cereals and breads, edamame, and soy milk. A good high-magnesium snack for Michelle would be whole-grain cereal and skim milk.
8. **Increase iron intake:** I recommend that Michelle add two iron-rich foods to her daily intake and consume them with a source of vitamin C—orange juice, for example—to help with the absorption of non-heme iron (iron from sources other than animal proteins). This should help with her energy, mood, memory, and concentration. It is possible that Michelle needs to take iron supplements, but we won't know until her ferritin level is checked.

9. **Add milk or fortified beverages for vitamin D and calcium:** Michelle should make sure she has at least two servings of milk or a fortified soy, nut, or rice beverage each day to help increase her vitamin D and dietary calcium levels. There are also calcium chews that are available for Michelle to try if she is open to that.
10. **Avoid or limit intake of caffeine, alcohol, and salt:**
    - Excessive intake of caffeine increases urinary calcium losses and is related to poor sleep and mood swings
    - Consumption of alcohol can contribute to hot flashes and night sweats, poor sleep quality, mood swings, and irritability.
    - Excessive salt intake is related to increased urinary calcium losses and increased blood pressure.
11. **Add vitamin D supplements:** Although we can aim to meet Michelle's iron, magnesium, and calcium requirements through diet, vitamin D should be supplemented. It is very difficult for an adult to meet his or her vitamin D requirements through diet alone. Vitamin D supplements are readily available in pill form, but because Michelle dislikes pills she can opt for the liquid form, which can also be given in weekly doses if she prefers. She should aim for 800 IU of vitamin D daily from supplements, and any extra she gets from food is still going to bring her intake in well below the tolerable upper intake of 4000 IU per day. An alternative would be to take 10,000 IU of vitamin D weekly or biweekly.

Follow-up visits

Follow-up visits were booked to help Michelle incorporate the nutrition plan into her daily life. At these appointments, I discuss techniques (including recipes) for incorporating soy and flax into Michelle's diet as she had never used these ingredients before, and I provide her with lists of high-magnesium and high-iron foods. I instruct Michelle on how to read and understand food labels. I assist her in modifying some of her favourite recipes by substituting healthier ingredients, then work with her to develop meal plans using these recipes. Finally, I evaluate Michelle's progress toward improving her health and minimizing her symptoms, and I make recommendations for future action.

Regina Kaiser, Meditation Teacher & Coach

Mendy pulled into the parking space, turned off the car, and closed her eyes. She needed a moment to collect herself.

Mendy liked to be on time. The drive through rush hour had taken longer than expected, and she was now late for her appointment. But instead of rushing in flustered, she decided it was better to take a moment to calm herself. This was, after all, a meditation centre, and she wanted to present her best self.

Mendy wasn't sure what was happening to her emotionally, mentally, and physically. Her kids were in their teens, and she was looking forward to spending more time with her husband as they became more independent. But she wasn't feeling like her usual self. Her mood changed from happy to annoyed in the blink of an eye, and bouts of depression were making it even harder for her to stay focused. The sleepless nights and occasional heavy or long menstrual cycles left her fatigued and stressed. Despite eating healthier and taking fitness classes four times a week, she was gaining weight and her clothes didn't fit comfortably anymore. Getting dressed was no longer enjoyable. There wasn't a lot of down time in her life, and it seemed like the more she tried to stay on top of things, the more they were slipping out of her control.

Mendy knew she was in perimenopause, and she wanted to get through this transition as naturally as possible. She knew she needed something new.

While searching Google for answers, she received a text from her best friend Karman: "Want to go for coffee?" It seemed Karman always knew exactly when to connect! It was on this morning in the café that Mendy noticed for the first time how incredibly calm and present Karman was. It seemed like no matter what was going on in her life, Karman was able to deal with things patiently. They'd known each other since their kids started elementary school, and they had shared many ups and downs over the years. Mendy knew Karman started meditating years ago after her mother died from cancer. She had watched and supported Karman, but Mendy didn't really relate to this approach. Mendy had tried meditating on her own once, but that only left her feeling more frustrated. She was a doer—more of an action person. Sitting still with her eyes closed just didn't seem productive to her. Mendy wondered, though, if she could find that "something" Karman had.

The much-needed coffee break, with a healthy dose of encouragement from Karman, brought Mendy to this moment sitting in her car with her eyes closed. Karman suggested the best place to begin was within. She explained there are different types of meditation, and that meditating with a teacher would help her get in touch with her own highest integrity so she could make confident and clear decisions in all areas of her life. Mendy realized she wanted a meditation that would allow her to meditate on her own and provide purpose, meaning, and results, just as Karman had done. Mendy smiled quietly, and for the first time in a long time, she felt hopeful. *Odd*, she thought, *I haven't even gone in yet and I already feel better.* She whispered, "Thank you Karman," and stepped out of the car.

Will and Intention

Mendy was ready for new beginnings, and she had a high level of commitment to healing and wholeness. The journey she began within through meditation required discipline and commitment. At first, Mendy resisted the idea of dedicating time she didn't think she had to meditating. However, her will and strong intuition kept her going.

Mendy understood it would take more than a couple meditation sessions for her to start feeling long-term benefits. She kept going to the meditation classes, and with a qualified teacher she discovered both shadow and light within her soul. Now, instead of avoiding the uncomfortable, she started to confront it and transform herself. She learned there would be times when she would question herself, and when she might feel like she was going backwards instead of forwards. She also learned there would be times she felt elevated to pure bliss, and her heart would be filled with joy. Both experiences are valid. By meditating regularly, Mendy was able to listen to her intuition in making conscious choices for the well-being of her whole self.

Boundaries

Prior to starting her meditation, Mendy noticed she had become more sensitive. She no longer wanted to be around negative or toxic environments. When she got home, she couldn't get work or other people off her mind, and she found herself tossing and turning in bed, unable to sleep. She started to avoid certain people and events that made her feel drained and exhausted. Her life was becoming limited, and she was tired all the time. She knew her physical body was changing, but she sensed there was more to learn.

In her meditation classes, Mendy discovered she was responsible for her own responses to people and events. She also learned that without boundaries, she was easily influenced by what other people thought was best for her. By establishing stronger energetic boundaries, she stopped blaming others for the way she felt. She cleared away her expectations and focused on her own healing. She learned to centre inwards and found a confident, clear voice to say "yes" or "no" as she needed to. She started feeling more alive and empowered in everyday life. Now, when she started noticing she was losing her space to others, she would centre inwards as spirit first. She started feeling more energized and calm, and people started noticing something "lighter" and clearer about her. She also started sleeping better.

Mendy continued meditating, and soon started to see the light at the end of the tunnel. She didn't have to give up wine or chocolate or other things in her life. Instead, she became more mindful and started celebrating each step of the way. She was more in touch with herself and her body, mind, emotions, and soul. She started taking time for her whole self by going to yoga and meditation regularly, eating mindfully, and spending time relaxing and having fun. When she started feeling overwhelmed in any area of her life, Mendy asked for help with a deep sense of clarity and trust.

Centring and Grounding

Mendy's decision to begin exploring meditation and mindfulness created a solid foundation of trust in herself and her life choices.

Mendy learned that when she is centred and grounded in the present moment, she is able to make clear decisions that reflect her own highest integrity; this is the first and most important lesson she learned. With continued practice, she started experiencing her essential nature as a peaceful spirit in a human body. She was able to identify her own needs, hear what others had to say, and respond with clarity and calm rather than reacting with fear. She became aware of her thoughts and feelings, but she was not as overwhelmed or controlled by them. She started relating to what and how her body was communicating with her. Even when she disagreed with another person, she was peaceful and able to share her perspective. Mendy's life became calmer and clearer, and her vitality increased.

With her new way of experiencing herself from within, centered and grounded in her body, Mendy realized there was so much more to meditation. She wanted to experience the changes in her body and life with greater awareness and enthusiasm. She now felt she could explore her options for balanced well-being with a greater sense of focus and stability.

Through meditation, Mendy discovered the most important relationship is the one she has with herself as spirit first. Her intuition, along with encouragement from her friend Karman to meditate with a qualified teacher, had given her the solid foundation she needed on her transformational journey through perimenopause, menopause, and the rest of her life.

Subtle Nuances

From early childhood, we have been taught to think about and experience ourselves through the external world. Chances are that as children, we were not shown how to look within or listen to our inner self. Imagine how a young girl might relate to the changes in her life if she was taught to trust her inner self and listen to her body, mind, and soul.

Excessive thinking, confusion, disappointment, worry, and seeking verification from others consumes vital energy and creates an imbalance between spirit, mind, body, and soul. For those with a racing mind, it is difficult to connect with the needs of the physical, emotional, and mental self. It is impossible to hear the wisdom within or the wisdom others have to share. With a changing physical body, it is imperative to calm the mind and emotions to reduce stress and anxiety so you can feel in control of your own well-being.

Women have been taught how to move and behave in the outer world, but many of us have limited training on how to trust our inner world and intuition. When a woman lives a busy life and her body is transitioning through physical, emotional, mental, and spiritual changes, it may seem impossible to find the time to turn inwards in stillness, especially if she has excessive thoughts. This is why the first and biggest obstacle to overcome is to trust that a disciplined meditation will guide her to inner stillness while calming the mind and relaxing the body.

Types of Meditation

The practice of meditation creates a direct path of awareness to nurturing spirit first, breathing for life, relaxing the body, and calming the mind. It allows a person to transform and transcend their thoughts, feelings, and physical discomforts while cultivating the intuitive process. Meditation brings a mindfulness that encourages awareness, acceptance, and focused clarity with relaxed calm.

Meditation is a precise technique, traditionally performed sitting upright with eyes closed, to attain a state of awareness that connects one to their core essence and infinite potentiality. However, there is no right or wrong way to meditate. Meditating while lying down encourages relaxation and sleep. Meditating while sitting still in an alert state, without any external distractions, encourages self-awareness, self-discovery, and transformation that brings mindfulness to everyday life, revealing the relaxed, confident, beautiful soul within.

Meditation is not a religion, but meditation may be used in some religious practices. You do not need to be spiritual or have anything wrong with you to meditate.

Today, thousands of people all over the world from every profession meditate every day, because they know it works. Most people are receptive and open to understanding how meditating works, especially as we discover which type resonates with our own personal needs.

Fortunately, "meditation" and "mindful" are words that have come to be used more extensively in our modern world. While there are different types of meditation, all support the individual in reducing stress and becoming calmer, clearer, and healthier. We have silent meditation, mindful meditation, relaxation meditation, conscious meditation, walking meditation, moving meditation, and more. A meditation can bring you either into your body or away from your body.

Meditation and yoga are a wonderful combination, although they are fundamentally different. Yoga is considered moving meditation and finishes with a peaceful, meditative pose known as savasana. You do not need to do yoga to meditate, and you do not need to meditate to do yoga.

For simplicity's sake, there are basically two types of meditation—relaxation/visualization and conscious meditation. Relaxation and visualization meditations offer short-term relief from anxiety, stress, and physical pain as they take you "away from" your body or reality for a short time. This type of meditation is usually offered in holistic therapies and at the end of a traditional yoga practice. However, when you return to your body, the discomfort and stress will eventually return; that's because when you arrive in the present moment, you realize your energy—as it relates to the physical, mental, and emotional bodies—has not changed much. It is similar to leaving a sink full of dirty dishes and going on a week's vacation, only to discover the dishes are still there and even dirtier than before you left.

For some, the temporary relief is more than enough. For those with an active mind, however, they may not be able to relax at all. They might find this type of meditation irritating and frustrating, leading them to believe that meditating doesn't work for them. In truth, though, they simply have not yet discovered the type of meditation that works for them. Additionally, how an individual feels and the life experiences they are moving through at the time they meditate will affect their experience. In all cases, it takes more than one session of meditation to experience long-term results.

A conscious meditation brings you into the present moment,

allowing you to be mindful and aware "in your body" and experience yourself as a peaceful spirit in a human body. This type of meditation is generally more disciplined as you centre inwards with present-moment awareness to uncover and heal all aspects of the mind, body, and soul. Conscious meditation is especially beneficial for an active mind as you do not need to stop your thoughts; rather, you learn how to stop letting them control you. This is also true for difficult emotions and the changes a person may experience in their life.

With practice and patience, the layers of conditioning that no longer serve you are cleared away and your true essence is revealed, allowing you to create and live a more peaceful life. You begin to feel relaxed, calm, and clear as you move through your day instead of seeking to escape the stresses of life.

In conscious meditations, you learn to be centred and grounded with boundaries, discovering compassionate ways to connect with your own needs alongside the needs of others. Through conscious meditation, you learn to be still and examine what is within yourself so you can attain the highest stillness and contentment, make confident decisions, and enjoy all aspects of your life...*all.*

Meditating takes patience and practice but does not need to take a long time. It is a healing process that creates wholeness and brings us together within ourselves and with others. Both relaxation/visualization and conscious meditations are beneficial in their own way, and they can be integrated together for an even richer experience. With a qualified teacher, anyone can learn to meditate, to transform judgment into acceptance, and to transform resistance into ease and flow.

Meditation is a personal journey inwards, and the most effective way to learn something is to experience it, not just read about it. People who meditate regularly are generally calmer, clearer, healthier, and have a more youthful demeanor. They manage difficult circumstances with a deep sense of trust and understanding. They have found the freedom to touch truth from within.

Women are intuitively drawn inwards to use their energy wisely, aligning their will with their intentions. However, the perception that they are in control is exactly that...a perception. When meeting the challenges of life head on, most women do not give themselves the time and energy they need to deeply feel and heal mentally, emotionally, physically, and spiritually. During the perimenopausal and menopausal stages, her soul brings awareness to the areas of life that need attention now, in preparation for the next phase of life. Her physical body is changing; she can either reject and fight these changes, or she can accept and embrace them.

At menopause, women have completed a rite of passage. On a soul level, this stage of life is an opportunity to surrender, let go, and trust the process. By doing this, a woman prepares herself to live life lighter and be ready to step into her next role.

Transformation through meditation and perimenopause is like the metamorphosis of the caterpillar into a butterfly. We do not know what or how we will feel during the transition, but we know we will emerge with wings to fly. Trust the process; begin within.

Dr. Angela Macdonald, Chiropractor

Are you stiff in the mornings? Does the thought of trying to run ten kilometres make you cringe while thinking about your sore hip? Do you find yourself rubbing your neck at the end of a day at the office and reaching for the Advil? Is it because you are getting old? Does this just happen with age, and are we powerless over the changes? I would like to challenge these thoughts and help rewrite the script of how you, and all middle-aged women, feel throughout the day.

I am so grateful that I chose to become a chiropractor—or, maybe life chose me!

You could definitely say that I am passionate about helping people make sure their physical body does not hold them back from what they're inspired to do in life. Whether that is being a mom or grandma, getting in eighteen holes on the golf course, painlessly travelling the world, finishing an Iron Man race, or maybe all of the above.

Unfortunately, in many cases people are held back from what they want to achieve due to back pain or headaches or hip pain. While I hate to say it, this awesome midlife adventure is when we often need a little more "maintenance"—or, shall I say, when the investment into a little more maintenance of our physical bodies has the most reward. This is where including a chiropractor in your life can be a huge benefit.

It is always interesting when someone asks me what I do in a social setting and I tell them that I am a chiropractor. They either tell me about how much they love their chiropractor, and then we discuss their shoulder issue for half an hour (fine with me, by the way—remember the passionate part?). Or, there is an awkward silence. I have had one person tell me that they don't believe in chiropractors—I felt a bit cheeky when I told him, "I am real."

So many people don't understand what we do, what our education is, and how we can help improve their lives. It is always fun to enlighten them and help them understand that, "No, once you go to a chiropractor you don't always have to go to a chiropractor." Many people choose to, though, because they feel like it adds quality to their life. They have chosen to be proactive with their body instead of reactive.

It is like going to a gym. If your goal is to lose ten pounds, you stay until you lose ten pounds. However, if your goal is to have good bone density and a healthy heart, then you might choose to make the gym a part of your lifestyle. Similarily, if your goal for coming to see me is to have no more pain in your shoulder, you will continue with care as we recreate proper shoulder mechanics until you have no more pain. If your goal is to maintain a supple spine even though you sit at a desk all day, you may decide to make your visits—along with daily exercises and stretches—part of your lifestyle. The important thing is that YOUR goals are listened to and respected, so make sure you find a chiropractor who does that.

All chiropractors start in first year physical science courses at university, along with future medical doctors, physiotherapists, and registered massage therapists. All of us know we want to go into a profession where we lessen suffering—we have many more commonalities than differences.

Depending on the chiropractic school, many students complete three to four years of an undergraduate degree before they can be accepted. Most people studying chiropractic medicine have a bachelor's or even a master's degree before starting their specific chiropractic training.

At the Chiropractic College or University, there are four more years of study where we go more in depth into anatomy, physiology, and biomechanics before learning about diagnosis, pathology, and actual adjustments and mobilizing techniques. We spend our last year studying and practising in student clinics. Once we graduate, we are allowed to use the title of "doctor" as we are trained to be able to decide, through a thorough history and exam, whether we can assist with the patient's problem or if we must refer them to other, more appropriate care.

People are often surprised to learn how many physical symptoms are related to our frame and how it moves and holds itself. Of course, everyone thinks of us helping back and neck pain—and we do have very good success with these problems—but a day in my office shows that we also have very good results with tension headaches, migraines, hip pain, shoulder pain, breathing restrictions, and athletic performance.

Some of the most rewarding patients to help are the moms who have always put everyone else first. They live with Advil in their purse for their chronic headaches or back pain, and they just manage their symptoms. If there has been no trauma to cause an injury, then often this mechanical back and neck pain comes from chronic postures and the weight of gravity pulling us down. If exercise is one of the things lost to a busy woman's schedule, then they have less core strength available to counter this gravitational pull.

Another situation that I see is the woman who makes time for her killer cardio workout, valuing the calorie burn and endorphin rush at the expense of stretching and core work. In this case, her muscles often get shorter and tighter, especially the ones on the front of her body (as is common with running and spin classes), which may already be shortened and tightened through hours spent at a desk job and/or in the car chauffeuring kids.

One of the most common complaints I hear from women in midlife is upper back and neck pain, often associated with headaches and fatigue. The secret to this discomfort, *which should not be a secret*, is that you have always had the power to feel better, even if you didn't know it—hello, Dorothy from the Wizard of Oz!

In many cases, this pain comes from gravitational stress through the joints, ligaments, and discs in your spine, as well as from muscles improperly pulling at the skeletal system. If you simply listen to the advice we all hear throughout our childhoods and "stand up straighter, for goodness' sake," many of these symptoms would self-resolve or never have been a problem in the first place. No one leaves my office without a talk about the power of posture.

When we allow ourselves to slump, our back goes into a "C" shape instead of the "S" shape that our spine *should* have. This puts a harmful load on our joints, compresses the discs between our vertebrae, and tightens our hip flexors which then puts strain on our pelvic and hip joints. And yes, all of that causes low back pain. Our shoulders also fall forward, and this puts a lot of stress between our shoulder blades, tightens the muscles through our chest, and shoots our head forward. Our head weighs ten pounds, and for every inch it goes forward, it puts an extra ten pounds of force on our neck—meaning that when our bodies are collapsed, our upper back and neck may be required to hold up the equivalent of fifty to sixty pounds. No wonder they get upset with us!

Back and neck pain are not the only issues than can result from poor posture. Try this at home: go ahead and let yourself slump forward and collapse, then try taking a deep breath. Hard, isn't it? Now sit tall like there is a helium balloon attached to your head and breath from there. Ah ha! Our breathing improves. All of our muscles, as well as our brain, need oxygen to work optimally; if we aren't getting enough oxygen, then it impacts our body's ability to function. As you can see with this experiment, when we are slumped forward we cannot breathe properly. So, while posture is not the only reason for a woman in midlife to be fatigued, it can certainly be a contributing factor.

So, the question that I most often receive from women, like you, who want more out of midlife is, "Do you think you can help me with my pain?" Often, this question will be attached to so much emotion, because women fear that my answer will be, "No, you are just getting old." I have seen too many vibrant, inspired eighty-year-olds for me to EVER give that answer. Yes, there may be some structural changes to your spine over the years, but in most cases the pain comes from unfortunate, slow-forming functional changes that we can alter by working together to correct them. I will always be committed if you are, although in some cases I may not be the professional you need to see most.

If it were you coming in to see me, my first step is always a thorough assessment, including learning your medical history and a physical exam. Once I've determined if your pain is an issue that I can assist you with, I would then explain that the pain pattern didn't happen overnight, so it won't miraculously fix it overnight either—although sometimes it actually does! I also would inform you that I will be responsible for some of your improvements, but you will also be responsible for making some of the changes that will last, which I will guide you through.

Sometimes, eliminating your pain requires inviting another member into your health care team. Maybe there is a food allergy creating extra inflammation in your body, so a naturopath would be helpful. Sometimes a tendon is irritated and requires work with an acupuncturist or a cortisone shot through your MD. There may be scar tissue in the muscles and connective tissue, requiring the skills of a registered massage therapist. Or, maybe you have played softball your whole life, resulting in a muscle imbalance from the rotation of your throw and batting swing, so you need a physiotherapist to rebalance the muscles involved. As you interview and choose the practitioners in your midlife health team, I recommend that you find out if they cross-refer with other professionals. In my option, if they say they can fix everything themselves, then you should be a bit leery.

If chiropractic care is brand new to you, then here is what a typical visit entails.

At a first visit, you will be warmly welcomed in a reception area and given some paperwork that will go over your current health challenges and your medical history. These are all important pieces of information for me to understand your body as a whole.

Once you are in my personal office space, I listen to your concerns and frustrations in your own words. We talk about how and why you think your pain or dysfunction started, what makes it worse, what makes it better, your job and hobbies, and your demands at home.

It is always helpful if you bring any previous x-rays, CT scans, MRIs, bone density tests, and joint-related blood work, along with a list of your medications. Within this information may be clues that allow me to help you more efficiently, know what treatments will be safest and most effective, and understand if there is too much risk in chiropractic care for you.

Next, I do an exam that involves seeing how your body holds itself while you stand. I will check for symmetry in your ear, shoulder, shoulder blade, and hip heights. I will watch the movement of your back, neck, shoulders, and hips. As the nervous system can be compromised by problems with the muscles and bones, I will check your reflexes (tap your knee, watch your leg kick up, and hear the giggle) and do other tests of the nervous system as required.

At this point I will lay you face down on the comfortable chiropractic table to assess the individual joint motion up and down your spine, looking for areas that are stuck or move too freely. I will also check the alignment of your vertebrae, see how tight and tender the muscles of your back are, and assess the symmetry of your pelvis and leg length. I will then have you turn face up and evaluate your neck. There are also area-specific tests I may do to locate the cause of symptoms such as headaches or shoulder pain. This whole exam is very comfortable; if anything, it feels a bit like a relaxing massage.

Once I have completed my assessment, you sit up and I describe what I found and let you know whether I think I can help or if there is someone else more appropriate to treat your symptoms.

Should we decide together that you are a good candidate for chiropractic care, we always review an informed consent sheet so you fully understand any risks associated with the suggested treatment. If you are still excited to go ahead and be partners on this journey, then we get started!

The actual chiropractic adjustments should not hurt. Sometimes, though, if we get something moving that hasn't moved in months or years, it can get a little sore for about forty-eight hours afterwards. The pain isn't horrible—it may feel like you have completed a tough work out—and ice really helps. Future appointments are tailored to your own specific circumstances, and I will often provide exercises for you to perform in between appointments.

One of the gifts of midlife is that as family responsibilities dwindle, we have more time for self-care. Once a woman decides to make herself a priority, there is instant empowerment as we review what is wrong, what my role is in her feeling better, and what her role is as well. As life's demands and priorities shift, that Advil in the purse is no longer needed, and she takes the energy that was once used up by the pain and puts it toward her relationships and career. Awesome!

As the mom of the house usually is in charge of the health care of her family, once she has experienced for herself how beneficial chiropractic can be, she often makes an appointment for her husband, who always groans getting out of bed in the morning after a hockey game. She makes another one for her daughter, the softball pitcher with the sore shoulder, and one for her son, who spends hours a day stooped over either his guitar or his phone. This means that one woman taking a step to improve her own health often has an impact on the people that she cares for the most!

While chiropractic care can make an incredible difference in reducing pain and improving function, what I want to be able to tell everyone is how important it is to avoid the poor habits that cause these issues from the get-go. The stronger your core muscles are and the more supported your trunk is, the less stress you place on the parts of your spine and pelvis that create pain. To help strengthen the core and stabilizing muscles of our body, Pilates—when done in small groups, with an educated instructor whose emphasis is on form—can be excellent. Yoga also has many poses that strengthen the core muscles and has the added bonus of flexibility training. More recently, I have become aware of Foundation Training (www.foundationtraining.com), which takes pieces from both Pilates and yoga and incorporates biomechanical and anatomy truths into a wise practise that complements any lifestyle.

Imagine a world where posture exercises and awareness were as much of a public health priority as washing our hands and brushing our teeth. Especially in this age of texting and excessive screen time, think of how much we could reduce back pain, neck pain, and headaches around the globe with this initiative. We can get over most infections and can get false teeth; our spines, on the other hand, cannot be replaced.

My last piece of advice is that as you approach any health care professional, ask what YOU can do. I think sometimes doctors believe that everyone is looking for the quick fix—prescriptions instead of nutritional changes to correct high cholesterol, antacids instead of mindful choices for heart burn, muscle relaxants instead of fixing the problems that caused the back pain in the first place.

As the wise Thomas Edison said, "The doctor of the future will give no medicine, but instead interest his patients in the human frame, diet, and the cause and prevention of disease." And as Albert Schweitzer said, "The doctor of the future will be oneself."

A good chiropractor will help you find this wise doctor inside of you.

Bob Mehr, Pharmacist

Shortly after I graduated as a pharmacist, I had a life-changing experience.

I was working at a well-known chain drug store in Prince Rupert, British Columbia. Now, you must realize that anyone who enters into a helping profession and dedicates a serious number of years to their studies, practicums, internships, and exams, eventually graduates with a very idealistic view of the world. I had devoted my life to learning about diseases and pharmaceuticals, conditions and treatments. I was armed with a big pile of information and naïve enough to think I was going to save the world.

So there I was in the real world, behind the counter in 1995, and I was on the telephone with a customer named Ron.

"How are you doing today?" I asked. It was a habit that has served me each and every day of the last twenty-two years.

"I'm not feeling well today," Ron replied from the other end of the telephone. "I need to have my ulcer medication refilled."

I chatted with Ron a bit more about what he was experiencing and suggested that if he wasn't feeling well, he should go see his doctor.

A few hours later, Ron was standing at the counter of my pharmacy with a prescription for his ulcer medication that he had just received from his GP. I didn't know it at the time, but what happened next would change the trajectory of my career as a pharmacist, as well as my life.

Ron's face began to turn blue, and then he collapsed to the floor. Minutes later, he died of a heart attack.

Our health care system had failed Ron. He wasn't educated on the signs of a heart attack, but he had taken my advice and gone to see his doctor, who had also missed the signs. Instead of getting the treatment he needed, he died in front of me with the prescription for his ulcer medication still in his hand.

You see, pharmacists have a much bigger role and responsibility beyond dispensing medication, counting pills, and telling people what to take, when to take it, and what side effects to watch for. Our role is to look after the whole individual in front of us; to be a resource for them, and to open the gates for them to access the health care and help they need.

The same month that Ron passed away, our store's targets had grown from filling 150 prescriptions per day to 160, from 4000 per month to 4500, all by one pharmacist and one technician and with even more pressure from head office to talk with every patient, discuss their condition, and provide them with the best counsel possible.

It became increasingly impossible to have a thorough conversation with patients when all my time was spent counting pills and updating the computer. I was lucky if I had thirty seconds with each person to tell them whether they should take their medication with food or on an empty stomach and review maybe two to three possible side effects.

This may not alarm you. You might be reading this and saying to yourself, "Yes, but isn't that what pharmacists do?"

Well, this is how consumers have been trained to think about the role of their pharmacist in their health. But as soon as I saw Ron lying on the floor of my pharmacy that day, I realized we play a much bigger role.

In survey after survey, pharmacists rank as one of the top-trusted professionals. However, many people don't realize that they can talk to pharmacists and tap into the depth and breadth of our education and expertise. Perhaps that's because we live and work mostly in a retail environment, and the unconscious assumption might be that we are sales professionals rather than health care professionals. I believe that if you can make this small but profound shift in how you think about the role of your pharmacist, it will help you to connect the dots of your own midlife health journey.

At our pharmacy locations, we encourage and invite our patients to come and talk to us. We are in constant communication with a large network of health care professionals and have established a culture of connectivity and collaboration; so if, perhaps, you need a chiropractor or a Reiki practitioner, we can make a recommendation or a connection that is best for you.

I am an integrative pharmacist who looks at the person as a whole. I do not push pharmaceuticals—I don't believe the answer to every health condition/disease/ailment is drugs. I have witnessed a lot of failure in the world of pharmacy and in the health care system, and all of them have pushed me to think outside of the box. This means not always following what my industry dictates or doing what has been traditionally done.

Pharmacists don't have the answer to everything. We are not doctors, naturopaths, physiotherapists, or energy healers. And yet, we need to know what expertise is available and what benefits can come from building a health team that includes all or some of these professionals. That way, when I am having a conversation with you about your health, I can help you decide who the best person is for you to see.

Knowing this, women have an opportunity to rethink how a pharmacist fits on their midlife health team.

Your pharmacist is one of the very few trained health professionals you can access without an appointment, and if we spend time with our patients, we have the opportunity to guide and direct them to the right outcome. We understand symptoms, conditions, medications, and their reactions and interactions. As an integrative pharmacist, I think about the whole patient rather than one-solution-per-problem. So, while I often address concerns with prescriptions, I am equally addressing exercise, diet, and supplements. I might be playing the role of counsellor or recommending a physiotherapist; I might also be suggesting my patients laugh more and find more joy in their lives. It's about seeing the person in front of me as a whole, and offering treatment as a whole.

Last week, a patient came in. She is very well educated and a health professional herself—she is a veterinarian. When I asked her "How are you doing today?" she smiled.

"Bob," she said, "whenever I come and see you, I start smiling. I may be in pain, but our conversations always make me feel better." She went on to explain that talking about her health choices, lifestyle tweaks, and even what she is doing in her life for fun leaves her feeling more confident that she is on the right journey and in control of her own health.

I founded my first integrative pharmacy in 1999. Our pharmacists are trained to fill both regular and compounded prescriptions in partnership with natural health advisors. Compounded prescriptions are where we custom-make the medication on site, which allows us to prepare medications to specifically match a patient's needs.

In the traditional pharmacy world, there are typically only one or two dosage forms as it is too complicated (or not as economical) to offer more choice. However, no two people are the same. Maybe you find it difficult to swallow pills and have been prescribed something that only comes in a large capsule format. As a compounding pharmacy, we might be able to prepare it as a liquid instead.

Our specialized training allows us to think about what the best way is to transport a medication into the patient's system. Sometimes that ends up being in pill form. Other times, it is via a transdermal cream, nasal spray, lozenge for under the tongue, or suppository. We do this to improve patient compliance, and to make sure the drug has the ability to do its job (which is called efficacy). These two things are very important for a successful health outcome for the patient.

For any prescription you bring in, we work to make sure the medication you are taking is the right medication for you. We want to understand why you are taking it, if you've tried anything else, and if you are experiencing any symptoms or side effects. If there are issues present, we probe to see if they are related to compliance, another condition, or even another side effect. We ask open-ended questions to help extract the full story or experience. And, because certain medications deplete our bodies of nutritional value, we can also recommend supplements or dietary changes to improve your intake of certain nutrients.

We encourage and invite our patients to come and talk to us. We are also in constant communication with a large network of health care professionals and have established a culture of connectivity and collaboration; so, if you need a chiropractor or a Reiki practitioner, we can make a recommendation or a connection that will benefit you.

During my first year of practice, I got married. My wife, Mahtab, is a pharmacist and co-founder of our company, Pure Pharmacy. That same year, I started seeing a somewhat vicious cycle with my female patients. The conventional, standard treatment for nearly every woman who had gone twelve months without a period, or who had reached the age of fifty or fifty-one, was an automatic prescription for estrogen (made synthetically from the urine of pregnant mares and branded Premarin) and synthetic progesterone (brand name Provera).

Often, these women would show up a few months later with a prescription for thyroid medication. And a few months after that, they would come back with a prescription for anti-depressants, and some would be back for anti-anxiety medication. It was a pattern I saw many times over, and I started to get concerned.

I began to do some research online. I read and read and read. I tried to learn whatever I could about bioidentical hormones. I consumed all of the books by Dr. John Lee, who was a renowned expert on hormone balance and authored numerous books on the subject, including *What Your Doctor May Not Tell You About Menopause*. What I was learning about bioidentical hormones just made sense to me; why were we giving women something that was not the same as what their bodies made?

I became intensely interested in this question, and in women's health. I took courses, attended seminars, and started helping my female patients. The results were positive. However, it was a challenging battle. I had pharmaceutical companies promoting synthetic drugs to me. I had physicians calling me asking why I was talking to their female patients about something the doctors knew little about. Despite these challenges, I was 100% committed. I had already witnessed a patient dying in front of me when my intuition was that medical intervention was required; I needed to follow my intuition in this scenario, too. I believed I could help to make a difference in the lives of my female patients—and in the lives of the men who love them!

Then came 2002, when the Women's Health Initiative (WHI) released its findings that women taking estrogen were at higher risk of certain cancers and heart disease. Researchers halted the WHI clinical trial altogether because of the noted increased risk. There wasn't a recall or a discontinuation of the therapy. However, with the news of the study making front-page headlines, women quit their hormone therapy cold-turkey, and doctors stopped prescribing the treatment because they did not want to be liable.

This was a really fascinating time for me, because some of the same doctors who had called me in the 1990's questioning why I was talking to their patients about bioidentical hormones were now calling to ask me what I could recommend for their patients. Their waiting rooms were now full of female patients experiencing hot flashes, night sweats, fuzzy thinking, anxiety, and sleep deprivation, and these doctors had limited options to offer.

Some doctors started prescribing specific anti-depressants to combat hot flashes. This is called off-labelling—when a drug intended and approved for one condition is prescribed for another. Consider all the women taking anti-depressants who are not/were not depressed as a result! Other doctors became curious and started to learn more about bioidentical hormone therapy, and they saw the benefits and positive health outcomes with their patients.

Over the last eighteen to twenty years, the battle certainly became a lot easier. I have seen a revolution and an evolution in the adoption of bioidentical hormone therapy, and I am so happy about it because now we don't have to watch our female patients suffer. Instead, we get to watch them celebrate and enjoy a quality midlife experience.

Many doctors and health professionals still have issues, particularly in answering two questions. The first one is, how can we prove bioidentical hormone therapy works?

The best way to answer this question is to look at the patient's experience. The women I see through our pharmacies are happier and have restored their quality of life, and they are not on any other medications. This tells us that the therapy is working.

The next question that arises is, how can we prove bioidentical hormone therapy won't cause breast cancer?

There has been no funding to prove whether or not bioidentical hormone therapy links to breast cancer. There have, however, been enough studies to support the idea that bioidentical hormone therapy is safe, so long as the patient is under the supervision of a qualified health care practitioner, they are on the lowest dosage for the shortest period of time to manage their symptoms, and an individual risk assessment of their family history of cancer is performed. As with any protocol, it is imperative for every patient to be monitored by their doctor and midlife health team for the duration of the treatment.

When the WHI results first came out, this risk made us all want to be on the safe side. After all, as pharmacists, we have taken an oath to do no harm. As time went on and more and more learning has occurred, it is in my professional opinion that bioidentical hormone therapy is safe. It is very individualized and depends largely on the woman herself. As long as she is under the supervision of a qualified health professional, and the bioidentical hormones are given at the right dosage and in the right format for her individual body, it is up to her and her doctor how long she stays on them. I have now seen some women (and men too!) take hormones into their late seventies and early eighties.

My personal experience has been that women who take bioidentical hormones report better quality of life, they are symptom-free, their lifestyle is better, their skin is improved, and their marriages are happier. Sometimes, I can see the improvement just by looking at them. However, I will be the first person to say that hormones are not everything. Rather, they are an option; a place to start in order to get the patient to begin to feel better. In a perfect world, we would start at the bottom of the health pyramid—with things like diet and sleep and lifestyle—and build up from there. There are no magic-wand solutions; hormone therapy is closer to a quick-fix, but the lifestyle foundation must still be present for there to be lasting results.

Positive health outcomes come through education and discussion. I had a recent conversation with functional medicine doctors about the idea of talking more openly about our health. When you think about it, conditions such as diabetes or cancer don't happen overnight; they are the result of a slow deterioration in health. So, if you transfer that thinking to women's health, we must start talking to women and educating them about their health at age eighteen or earlier. I have two daughters who are fifteen and eighteen, and my wife and I have a responsibility to talk with them and pay attention to their periods, moods, and overall lifestyle and health. I invite you to do the same with your children. Talk about the birth control pill, and be aware of the consequences it can have. I'm not against the birth control pill;

however, I am all for being informed and educated about the effects it can have on the body, and even how it can impact your transition through midlife.

Education is the most important ingredient to a smooth transition. I would even recommend starting a health binder and tracking everything you can. If possible, have your hormone levels checked when you are in your late twenties or early thirties; this is typically when health is optimal for most women. We all function differently with different levels of hormones. Your low could be someone else's high, and somebody's high could be someone else's low. Tracking allows you to refer back to what your previous levels were, and which helps us ensure we are not over-dosing or under-dosing you with hormones; we only need to bring you up to the level where you are functioning and feeling your best.

By far the most common conversation I have with women is they will say something like "I'm just not feeling my best" or "I feel so drained" or "I have no interest in sex any more" or, particularly over these last few years, "I think my iron is low." It's hard for them to pin point their exact pain, but overall, they know their quality of life isn't where it could or should be.

If a woman is in perimenopause (between age thirty-nine and fifty-five), there are also easy recommendations to make such as supplementing with a good quality vitamin B complex and supporting the adrenals with good quality sleep, napping in the afternoon, and practicing relaxation rituals such as yoga, meditation, walking in nature, and taking hot baths. Eating well, exercising regularly, and ensuring there is strong social support and lots of laughter in her life are also incredibly important. If her iron levels are truly low, then an iron supplement will often give positive results in a short amount of time.

Depending on the conversation, we might also recommend magnesium (restores energy and helps with sleep; most adults are deficient because it is hard to get adequate quantities from diet alone), rhodiola (reduces stress-related fatigue, improves mental performance and concentration, decreases cortisol levels and depression), ashwaganda (reduces anxiety), vitamin C (restores cortisol production), or other specific supports that are best matched to the woman's health goals or concerns. Always consult with a professional before beginning a new supplement. You don't need to navigate the vitamin aisle alone; get recommendations from an experienced professional who can explain what is going to work best for you.

This advice applies to anyone being proactive with her own health, regardless of age or condition: before you start any therapy, be sure to educate yourself and learn about your body and your cycle. Once you have that information, you can make a decision that is right for you through consultation with your health care professional. This is especially helpful in empowering women to be their own best health advocates. When empowered and informed women come up against a neighbour who says, "Maybe it's all in your head," they can turn around and confidently say, "I know I am not crazy; I know it is about hormone balance, and I am making informed decisions about my own health!"

Twenty-first century medicine is about information and empowerment. Empowerment comes with intention, so when you set out with good intentions, what you choose will most likely work for you. The moment you have doubt, the treatment is likely going to stop working. Educate yourself, look at the science, and look at the evidence. Empower yourself as the captain of your midlife health team, and invite family members and friends who care about you to join your team too.

Speaking of teams, one of the biggest myths about perimenopause, in my opinion, is that as a woman, you need to tough it out; that it's "normal" and you must put up with it. And you know what happens in perimenopause? Moods go up and down. Anxiety goes up and down. Libidos go up and down. Communication naturally goes down or disappears, and our relationships end up suffering; most divorces happen in this life phase. So, I invite you to educate yourself first, and then educate your partner and your children. Make them an essential part of your health team. As a husband, the more I know, the more I can understand. I have learned not to take any of my wife's experiences personally, and that there are changes going on in a women's body that I couldn't begin to fathom. I can empathize, but only with education and information.

Remember: there is no magic solution. The only magic is in empowering yourself.

Case Study: Rebecca

Rebecca is fifty-three, and she walked into our Pure Pharmacy location in West Vancouver back in 2015 with symptoms of fatigue, low energy, hair loss, feeling cold, weak and brittle nails, and brain fog. Many of these symptoms can be indicative of low thyroid function or hypothyroidism, and some of the symptoms can also be related to perimenopause or menopause.

Background:

Low iron is one of the most common things I see in women who walk through our pharmacies on daily basis. It's also one of the most common tests doctors run, and they do this by looking at ferritin levels (a measure of iron stores in your body). The normal reference range for ferritin is anywhere from 10-291 ng/mL for women. Most often, if women are not clinically anemic and their ferritin is within this range, doctors won't be alerted to abnormal ferritin levels (even if they are as low as 15, for example). However, recent studies show that women have improved energy and feel best with ferritin levels that are greater than 55 ng/mL, even if they are not anemic.

Women are more likely to have low iron levels than men, and they are also more likely to have hypothyroidism or Hashimoto's Disease. People don't usually think of iron as being essential to thyroid function, but it is!

The next steps:

With this in mind, the first thing I asked Rebecca to do was to ask her doctor to check her ferritin level and her thyroid function. A week later, she came back and told me that her doctor said her ferritin level was 7 ng/mL, and she urgently needed to start iron supplementation. Her tests showed her thyroid was also low, and she was given a prescription for thyroid medication.

A common issue with iron supplementation is that it can cause a lot of stomach irritation and constipation, which will lead some women to skip doses or stop taking it entirely. However, there are some iron supplements which are easier on the stomach and do not cause too much constipation. I gave her one of my own formulations which I developed back in 2001 because it is easy on stomach and has a very low side effect profile while still delivering enough elemental iron to bring ferritin levels up. She started taking one capsule every morning.

Within three weeks, Rebecca came back to report she was feeling great again, her energy level was much better, and she had noticed her hair was not falling out as much. She continued taking the iron for another six months, and eventually her ferritin level went up to 65 ng/mL. At that point, the recommendation for her was to continue checking her ferritin level every six months to ensure she was getting enough iron, and to monitor her thyroid function. She is now a regular patient at the pharmacy and is in good health.

What Should Your Ferritin Be?

For optimal energy and thyroid function, ferritin levels should be at or above 80 ng/mL. Hair loss or hair thinning can occur at levels less than 40. Anything below 30 is what I call "scraping the bottom of the iron bucket." If your ferritin is really low, your thyroid won't function properly no matter what other medications or supplements you are taking. Most women I see have ferritin levels somewhere between 20-50 ng/mL, and many are in need of some sort of iron support or supplementation.

That said, we also don't want too *much* iron, as this can be harmful to the body. Supplement wisely and make sure to re-test your levels on a regular basis.

Keep in mind that many symptoms of iron deficiency and hypothyroidism overlap. What you thought were low thyroid symptoms (such as fatigue and hair loss) could in fact be due to low iron! Your thyroid requires adequate iron levels to activate two key enzymes that are vital to hormone production and activation. If you have low thyroid function or hypothyroidism, have your ferritin levels assessed and get a copy of the results. Use 70 ng/mL as a guide to optimal levels, although different people feel best at different levels.

If you experience heavy menstrual periods, are vegan/vegetarian, or have digestive disorders that affect nutrient absorption (such as celiac disease), it's also important to have your ferritin assessed on a regular basis. Ask your doctor about testing your ferritin levels, and if needed, ask your pharmacist for the best iron supplements to increase your levels quickly without causing digestive upset.

Dr. Bal Pawa, Integrative Physician and Pharmacist

Shirley asked me what the one thing is that I want women to know about perimenopause. My answer, given that I spend a significant part of each day talking to women about hormones, surprised her.

I said, "At the turn of the last century, women lived to be fifty. Menopause was a non-event. Now, women expect to see their hundredth birthdays and beyond—yet, retirement communities and nursing homes are filled mostly with women, many who are challenged with osteoporosis and dementia-related conditions." It is not enough for us to have quantity of life, we must aspire to have quality of life as well.

The message I want every woman to understand is that hormone balance is only one slice of the midlife health pie. It is important. Whether you experience symptoms on your perimenopause-to-menopause journey or not, ALL women must pay attention to their whole health at midlife if they want to set themselves up for longevity and vitality. What we do now will have a significant impact on our quality of life in the second half of our journey.

After obtaining my degree in pharmacy and then graduating from medical school in 1988, I started practicing in Burnaby, BC. Right from the start, I saw a lot of female patients with a focus on gynaecology and obstetrics. During that time, I discovered many women were not going for regular Pap tests, particularly if their family doctor was male.

Together with one of my colleagues, we spearheaded a Pap clinic through the Vancouver Health Board to combat this issue. The clinic allowed women to be tested regularly while still keeping their family doctors.

It's been a long journey from then to now. As I look back, I realize it was those early practice days and the Pap clinic experience that really fueled my passion for women's health.

Women are the cornerstone of healthy communities. When we can keep women healthy or get them back on their feet after an illness or a period of not feeling well, it has a great impact on the health of our society at large. That's because women are our nurturers, conveners, and caregivers, and in many families they are also key providers. Women love to share information and help each other. I enjoy being part of their journey by giving them good credible information to share with their friends and family.

I co-founded the Westcoast Women's Clinic for Hormone Health as a result of my own personal experience. While I was navigating my own perimenopause journey, I had been in a bad car accident that left me with chronic pain and insomnia. These experiences compounded the hormone changes I was already noticing. Trying to be proactive and reactive with both these situations at the same time meant I had to quickly learn how to be an advocate for my own health. In doing so, I went on to receive certification from the Mind-Body Institute at Harvard Medical School. This was transformative to my career, it made me realize the importance of stress hormones on almost every system in the body including women's ovaries.

When a doctor can't find answers to her own health questions, it's a problem! It was confusing and frustrating, and navigating hormone health was particularly challenging for me with so much controversy in the news at the time.

You see, I did know where to look and who to ask to best guide my perimenopause experiences. It was just that their answers all included medication and pharmaceuticals, and none of those felt like the right option for me. There was a distinct lack of options for women, like me, who wanted to approach midlife health from a more holistic perspective.

It was around that time that I met Dr. Nishi Dhawan, and together we formed the Westcoast Women's Clinic in 2002. We were the first physician-based clinic in British Columbia to be fully dedicated to hormone health and wellness. We both became board certified through the North American Menopause Society (NAMS) and continue to stay up-to-date on the newest research on hormone therapy by attending regular conferences and educational events. Dr. Shannon Trainor joined the clinic a few years ago and is also a NAMS-certified menopause clinician.

As has been discussed previously in this book, the early 2000s was a turbulent time for both medical professionals and our female patients. The Women's Health Initiative (WHI) had just released its damning report on hormone replacement therapy (HRT), and women were told they had to stop taking hormones out of fear of increased risk for certain cancers, heart disease, blood clots, and other conditions. It was front-page news. This came after decades of doctors prescribing HRT to nearly all women who presented with complaints related to menopause—and sometimes even to those women who didn't complain, but who had reached a certain age. Now doctors were told to stop prescribing and women were told to stop taking hormones. Many women quit cold turkey without tapering off their hormones, or without any alternative or back-up plan to manage their symptoms. Many ended up on sleeping pills and anti-depressants.

As a trained pharmacist, I knew that hormones were important to health but the route of delivery for hormone therapy was equally important. The estrogen hormones that had been prescribed to women during this time were from a *natural* source—that natural source being the urine of pregnant mares. But Premarin (a name derived from PREgnant MARes' urine) is not molecularly equivalent to the hormones produced by a woman's body. When women take Premarin orally, the hormones pass through the liver, which has a very complex enzyme system that breaks down whatever you feed it. Oral estrogen goes through the liver and forms proteins in the blood which thicken the blood and result in a higher chance of strokes and blood clots. In fact, even oral contraceptives which are synthetic estrogens, have a higher chance of forming blood clots.

So, as we were launching Westcoast Women's Clinic, we decided we would only use transdermal estrogen (applied to the skin which penetrates into the bloodstream) and natural progesterone with our patients. We started with scientific hormone measurement, an individual risk assessment and at the lowest dose possible. We did a very comprehensive assessment of each patient detailing their exact symptoms and experiences, their severity, all of the potential risks, and whether or not the patient needed hormone therapy at all or if there was another protocol that could achieve the desired results.

As a physician and a woman in perimenopause, I had to take care of myself through my own journey. When it came to the question of whether hormone therapy was the right option for me, I needed to choose carefully. Through consultation with my primary health care provider, and through weighing the benefits versus the potential risks, I chose the lowest possible dose and transdermal (skin) route for estrogen. I also chose molecularly identical estrogen as opposed to synthetic. If a woman has a uterus she must also take progesterone to protect its lining.

It's ironic that as I write this in late 2017, the news has just been released that hormone therapy has been deemed safe on an individualized basis, as long as all of the precautions I took, including a comprehensive risk assessment and regular monitoring, are part of the physician's prescribed protocol. A lot of women between 2002 and today, who could have been candidates for hormone therapy, may have suffered unnecessarily due to misinformation and fear.

Many people wonder how a private clinic works in Canada when we have universal health care. When we first opened, we used the Medical Services Plan (MSP) model, which allows doctors to bill the government for a five- to twelve-minute appointment for every symptom. As you know, women's health is far more complex. The conversations with our patients were long, hormone therapy was (and continues to be) controversial, and a lot of our appointment time was spent educating, evaluating risk, and discussing priorities with women who presented with multiple health concerns.

We asked the College of Physicians to work with us on an integrative approach. We asked if we could provide education, health coaching, and comprehensive care for all hormones, even stress hormones—not just estrogen and progesterone—because hormones don't work in isolation; they all talk to one another. The response was if we were treating a medical issue, the College would pay for it. But if we were providing education or preventative care they would not, nor would they pay for hormone testing.

As much as we boast about our awesome health care in Canada, it has been built on a reactive sickness model, and we wanted to create a proactive wellness model for women. It was unique to offer this outside of the traditional medical model, but women were demanding support for their perimenopause-to-menopause journeys. We pushed forward and mandated that both education and empowerment be part of our clinic's mission, as we wanted women to make health decisions based upon good, credible information. We created a multidisciplinary team that includes a nurse educator, herbalist and kinesiologist, as well as connections to psychologists, physiotherapists and nutritionists.

We created a hybrid model with testing and lifestyle coaching paid by the patient, and treatment of medical conditions and necessary tests i.e. Pap smears and breast exams, paid by MSP.

In recent years, we partnered with like-minded physicians at Balance Medical Centre in Vancouver, an integrative medical clinic with naturopathic and medical doctors. This relationship has confirmed our conviction that a collaborative, team-based model is the most effective way to educate and empower women to take charge of their health. We are a practice of women working for women, and as such we are evidence that the best answers come from two or more minds working together.

This path has led us to the launch of a new integrated model for women's health (fall 2018) where women are cared for by a team including a patient educator, a NAMS-certified medical doctor and a doctor of naturopathic medicine. This is similar to how our clinic has been serving women over the last seventeen years, except the addition of a naturopath to the care team removes the question women often have about hormone health: "Should I see my doctor or should I see a naturopath?"

Working with the West Coast Women's Clinic

We call this new patient experience an annual health plan. Initially, a new patient talks to our patient educator and completes an intake form and a confidential personal health questionnaire so we know your health history, including but not limited to, your most recent Pap, mammogram, last period, and last blood work. We invite women to attend a workshop for education around hormones and how they work.

At the first appointment, women consult with both a medical doctor and a naturopathic doctor. Based on her risk assessment and her individual needs, the doctor may prescribe hormones at the first visit, or she may recommend that the patient complete a Comprehensive 24-Hour Urine Hormone Panel first. This hormone panel is our preferred method of testing as it is the most comprehensive in order to understand hormone levels and the body's ability to metabolize hormones. The doctor will check or discuss things like blood pressure, thyroid, heart health, breast health, and give a pelvic exam, if required. The medical doctor will also discuss a treatment plan at this time, which could include a conversation about hormone therapy.

Then the patient consults with the naturopath on her health team. This meeting reviews diet and lifestyle, options for administering the prescribed treatment plan, discusses key health goals and next steps.

The second appointment is a three-way consultation between the medical doctor, the naturopath and the patient. Navigating hormone health can sometimes take between four-to-fourteen visits in the first year or two. It's important we create an environment where a woman's health is regularly reviewed by her health team and any necessary tweaks or adjustments can be discussed and administered efficiently.

Outside of these appointments, the medical doctor and naturopath consult together on your particular case. That means, your care team is meeting outside of your appointment time to review and discuss any unusual or exceptional circumstances, or to simply provide updates. We know from past experience that this type of dialogue amongst care teams produces better (and quicker) health outcomes for women in our clinic! And the whole experience results in a very personalized health experience for the patient.

We work on an annual fee model which some extended health insurance plans cover. This is encouraging and has certainly evolved over the years. We like to give insurance providers a very comprehensive account of what we did and what protocols were recommended as we believe it helps to create change for the future of extended health benefits and move the dial closer to ensuring more women have access to the support they require.

To prepare for your first visit, bring a copy of whatever health records you have: Pap results, mammogram, blood work, and past medical history. Prepare for a lot of personal questions as we ask about libido and vaginal atrophy. We also encourage you to bring in all of your own questions too; no question is off-limits.

Common Concerns

We see a lot of women with mild, moderate, and severe symptoms, ranging from hot flashes, night sweats, insomnia, fatigue, depression, vaginal dryness, painful intercourse and weight gain. Sometimes women come for painful fibroids. The earlier you come in, the better; the longer it's left, the more intervention will be required. If you are in pain, or the fibroid is pressing against your bladder, it may be too late to avoid surgery. However, if they are small and caught early, there's a good chance we can do something less invasive. That might include progesterone plus a diet that's low in fat and includes iodine (such as sea vegetables and kelp), which helps to convert estrone (inflammatory estrogen) into estriol. There are also preventative strategies we can explore, depending on the size or stage of the fibroid.

We work with women after they have had a hysterectomy. Sometimes, we will see evidence of fragmented care—such as a woman who hasn't been offered any hormone therapy or been told what to expect post-surgery. If the ovaries have been removed, then this can be a bigger problem. If the woman's uterus was removed but her ovaries still function, she may reach ovarian failure faster/reach menopause sooner than she would have otherwise. In either case, hormone therapy might be a consideration—one that is best discussed before the surgery occurs.

Probably the most common conversation we have at the clinic is: Are hormones safe? As mentioned above, the answer is very individualized; there is no one-size-fits-all solution, it is a risk/benefit analysis.

In addition to evaluating family history during our risk assessment, we must also consider the following before beginning HRT:

- **Smoking:** If I meet a woman who smokes and lives a very sedentary lifestyle, I may not prescribe hormone therapy.
- **Alcohol:** Daily alcohol consumption is an irritant to the brain

and a contributor to breast cancer. It's riskier than hormone therapy.

- **Family history of breast cancer:** Although hormones do not cause breast cancer, we avoid them in patients with breast cancer. We choose non-hormonal treatment instead. A family history of dementia, heart disease, diabetes, stroke, depression and osteoporosis are also important genetic factors to consider.
- **What is the best mode of delivery:** Oral versus transdermal.
- **What is the optimal dosage:** Generally speaking, we say low-dose, transdermal hormone therapy is safe, but you must be specific with each case.

Hormones work like a lock and key with the receptor on our tissues. Our bodies have all these receptors crying out at menopause because the hormones have declined sharply. They were used to getting estrogen and progesterone, but now low levels are causing uncomfortable symptoms. The first eighteen months after your last menstrual period is when you should take hormone therapy, as this is when the biggest loss of bone occurs. Timing is very important. When physicians prescribe hormone therapy, they are not giving it at the same levels as your body would make it naturally. When you are ready to stop taking hormones, we decrease or taper the dose so you go through a very natural cessation.

As for the length of treatment, we used to say five years. Now, the latest positioning statement from the North American Menopause Society says ten years, which could be until a woman is sixty or sixty-five. But again, treatment plans must be individualized. If a patient has a higher risk for cancer, heart disease, or other chronic health conditions, I would have her come off of hormone therapy sooner rather than later. Women who have more benefit—let's say they have a higher risk for osteoporosis or they have dementia in their family—may benefit from staying on it until they are sixty-five. The bottom line is that hormone therapy protocols must be monitored regularly with your doctor/health care professional.

What Your Doctor Learned at Medical School

Some women feel dismissed by their physicians. They hear things like "you're just getting older," "you'll get through it," and "you'll be fine."

If you think about a doctor's paradigm for a minute, you will realize that society has let us—and them—down. I teach medical students at the University of British Columbia (UBC), and I can assure you that it is not that doctors don't care; it's that doctors are educated based on problem-based, or disease-based, learning. Menopause is not a big topic in medical school because it is not a disease. It does get covered as a sub-section in the endocrinology unit and is presented as a milestone in a woman's reproductive cycle in the gynaecology section. But, there is little focus on the experiences of the perimenopause-to-menopause journey. They may learn how to prescribe hormone therapy, but not much time is devoted to the prevention of symptoms or the impact on quality of life. In order to get that education, doctors must invest their own time and resources; if medical students show interest in women's health, UBC does have a women's health specialty for family doctors. I'm hopeful the standard curriculum will change to include more information on this topic, but it takes time.

With this in mind, it's easier to understand how a family physician must struggle. He or she has a waiting area full of patients. In one treatment room there is someone with an asthma attack, in another there is a person reporting chest pain, and in the third treatment room there's a baby crying. All three are triaged as urgent care. Women seeking information and care for hormone changes fall through the cracks—even when their experiences (lack of sleep, hot flashes, anxiety, depression, pain with intercourse) are debilitating.

It's important to make women aware of what each health care provider has in his/her toolkit. We can't assume our physicians have been educated in perimenopause/menopause or received additional certification in that area. Some have; some have not. It's okay to ask!

Some doctors who are not current on hormone therapy will refer patients to our clinic.

The following two case studies are success stories because, like many of my patients, they came to me ready to take action and be active members of the physician-patient care team. We are delighted to meet patients who are ready to partner with their doctor, because we are passionate and educated. But, it takes a patient who is motivated and committed in order for our "team" approach to work.

Case Study: Kathy

I met Kathy when she was forty-two. She was a successful realtor who also supported her husband with his busy renovation business. A high achiever with a remarkable ability to "cope" with whatever life threw her way, Kathy arrived in my office almost at wit's end. She complained of being irritable and experiencing unmanageable, angry outbursts towards her kids and her husband. She had noted in her day planner that the outbursts seemed to be much worse ten to fourteen days before her period. Kathy was also experiencing night sweats a couple of days before her period but didn't think too much of it, even though it was interrupting her sleep. She told me she was having headaches for the first time in her life, and her period was heavier than it used to be.

I asked Kathy a series of lifestyle questions and learned she smoked ten to fifteen cigarettes a day and usually drank three cups of coffee each morning. She exercised occasionally but found it hard to squeeze in amongst her stressful and demanding job and her kids' schedules.

Kathy came to see me because her sister suggested she may be feeling this way due to fluctuating hormones. Her first question was whether or not she is too young for perimenopause.

I explain the roller coaster ride also known as perimenopause; how estrogen peaks, but that sometimes progesterone can't keep up with it.

As a result, women often experience breast tenderness, cramping, and PMS in the luteal phase (last two weeks of her cycle). I also explain that some women will experience a more severe roller coaster if they have a poor lifestyle.

In Kathy's case, we did not immediately jump to hormone therapy. Instead, we chatted about the benefits of stress management and exercise and the downsides of sleep deprivation and smoking. I encouraged her to try taking melatonin and reducing her sugar, caffeine, and alcohol intake as well as her smoking. We decided to test her hormones, including her cortisol.

When the tests came back, her cortisol was very high, her progesterone was very low, and her estrogen was quite dominant (as was also evidenced by her sore breasts, heavy period, and clotting). I shared her test results with her, which showed Kathy was "tired-yet-wired."

I explained how she is wired because her stress is so dominant that it's pushing on her cortisol pathways. As a result, her adrenal glands can't keep up with the demand, so they are starting to steal progesterone from her ovaries to compensate.

Our goal was to get Kathy's hormone "symphony" under control. My first recommendation was to try taking evening primrose oil, vitamin B, and magnesium, but this wasn't enough to right Kathy's ship. We added 20 mg of progesterone cream for the last two weeks of her cycle, and Kathy reported back that this helped immensely.

I wanted Kathy to understand that she didn't have to quit her job, but that her stress hormones were at their maximum. We discussed self-care, relaxation techniques, and ways to set boundaries.

When I saw Kathy three months later, her condition had improved significantly. She had had a heart-to-heart with her husband and her teenagers. Her PMS was better, and she was down to three cigarettes per day. The progesterone therapy was helping with her bleeding and she was no longer anemic.

Case Study: Anna

I met Anna when she was fifty-four and running her own wellness centre. Her last period was three years go. Her family doctor had prescribed oral Estrace, which is a natural, bioidentical estrogen, but she had stopped taking it due to the conflicting controversies she had heard about hormone therapy in the media.

Since then, she had tried herbal remedies, black cohosh, and acupuncture. Her primary ongoing complaints were foggy brain, insomnia, pelvic pain, vaginal dryness, and bleeding with intercourse. Anxiety and hot flashes had also started to make an appearance, and she felt that her quality of life was dropping.

Anna was under a lot of stress. Her aging mom wasn't well, her marriage had dissolved recently, and her son had been managing his mental illness poorly.

Anna was at a healthy weight, didn't smoke, drank three to four glasses of wine per week to help her relax, and exercised and practiced yoga daily. She had a family history of osteoporosis, and her risk for heart disease was high. She was already wary of hormone therapy before we began.

We performed some testing, along with a thorough risk assessment. Her tests showed her estrogen and progesterone were both low, while her FSH was very high. DHEA was low. Testosterone was low. Cortisol was low.

Anna's lifestyle was good. She could maybe reduce the amount of wine she was drinking, but her blood pressure was good, as was her cholesterol and stress management. Her estrogen ratio quotient was also pretty good, which is an important part of any risk assessment for breast cancer.

I explained her risk assessment, as well as the latest research on hormone therapy, and recommended to Anna that she might benefit from hormone therapy. I performed a complete physical and sent her for a mammogram. I recommended that she take estrogen transdermally because she was still only three years out from menopause—had she been ten years out, I wouldn't have put her back on estrogen as I wouldn't want to wake up those breast cells. I also prescribed bioidentical estrogen, Prometrium (the brand name for oral micronized progesterone) at bedtime, and some compounded estriol vaginal cream to remedy her vaginal dryness (something that is important to address as it will not get better on its own.) We stressed the importance of vitamin D and calcium in her diet as well resistance straining to keep her bones strong. We also ordered a bone density test.

When I saw Anna three months later, her hot flashes had diminished, she was sleeping better, her brain fog had cleared, and her vaginal dryness had improved significantly. She no longer had pain with intercourse, and she was starting a new relationship. When I asked her how she felt and what she thought of her current health plan, she said that the speed at which her symptoms improved was much faster than she thought it would be. She was pleased she did not have to take multiple drugs such as sleeping pills and antidepressants for her symptoms. Anna was very grateful that we were taking steps to prevent osteoporosis, continued on her hormones safely and enjoys an excellent quality of life.

Dr. Cobi Slater, Doctor of Natural Medicine

My first introduction to natural medicine came at a very young age. My mom always had a strong belief in the healing power of natural medicine remedies and sought them first whenever I needed treatment for any health issues. My grandpa was an herbalist, and I witnessed him using herbal remedies to treat common ailments throughout my life. It was their belief systems that instilled in me a strong confidence in natural medicine.

I knew early on that I wanted to be a doctor or a pharmacist. I can remember being fascinated when I would see people telling the pharmacist their symptoms, and then he would go and make a remedy to help them. I would often wonder why these people had these symptoms and what was causing them. My inquisitive nature would take over as I wanted to understand the "why" underneath what they were experiencing. This curiosity is what eventually led me to become the type of practitioner who always treats the underlying causes rather than just dealing with the symptoms.

In 1994, my mom became seriously ill with a rare blood disease. At the time, I was completing my Bachelor of Science as I was planning to become a conventional physician. Over the course of the following year, my mom was in and out of the hospital and clinically died three times, thankfully being brought back to life each time! Without the help of conventional medicine, I would not have my mom today. However, after months of treatments, she was as stable as she could be and was released to go home. The prognosis was for her to remain on bed rest with limited activity for the rest of her life. My mom returned home but did not remain in bed; rather, she sought out natural doctors, who helped her completely regain her health! Witnessing this, I knew that I needed to switch my field of study into natural medicine.

All of this led me to become a doctor of natural medicine, clinical nutritionist, and medical herbalist. I also have a Ph.D. in Natural Health Sciences, with a specialty in endocrine dysfunction (hormone conditions). I chose this route of education so that I could experience the most in-depth training in each of the modalities I was interested in, including herbal medicine, nutritional medicine, therapeutic orthomolecular nutrition, supplementation, and endocrine dysfunction. It took me thirteen years of schooling to complete all of this.

Hormones are basically an intricate symphony that happens in the body. Imagine an orchestra; if one of the instruments is suddenly out of balance or out of tune, then that is going to throw off the entire group! They need to play together in perfect unison for everything to sound beautiful. Hormones are the same. They basically act like a highway of communication, allowing the different parts of the body to talk with one another. If there is a breakdown in the communication because the hormones are out of balance, the resulting ripple effect can literally occur in any part of the body and cause a variety of symptoms.

There is a dramatic increase of women experiencing hormone dysfunction in our society, which can create a plethora of symptoms. The underlying causes are often overlooked or undiscovered, and people are prescribed medications that simply mask their symptoms and ultimately do not offer a cure.

Hormone imbalances can occur very quickly or very slowly. For example, the thyroid commonly goes out of balance after childbirth, but the symptoms are often overlooked and blamed on being a new mother. Alternatively, some hormone imbalances develop over many months or even years, like a dimmer switch slowly going down. Many women do not notice this change; or, if they do, they choose to ignore the symptoms due to their hectic lives. Over a period of time, women start to notice that they don't have as much energy as they used to, or that they are finding it more difficult to lose weight than before. Mood swings can become increasingly challenging, sleep becomes a thing of the past, and PMS can start to feel never-ending.

Hormone imbalances can also show up in the form of stress. The stress in our life is cumulative, and there is a threshold for what we can handle. Picture a cup, and stress as water being poured into it. Slowly, the water level becomes higher and higher until it reaches the top. At this point, any extra stress will cause the cup to overflow. Often women will think, *These things did not bother me before. I used to be able to just roll with it. What is wrong with me?*

Excessive stress can show up in the form of anxiety or insomnia. Abdominal weight gain is also very common when we have high levels of stress; the receptors for our stress hormones are highly concentrated in our midsection, and as increasing amounts of the stress hormone cortisol is produced, the fat storage effects of this hormone take over the body.

Many other symptoms of stress and hormone imbalance can plague women, such as irritability, headaches, and skin changes like eczema, adult acne, or even rapid aging. Some of the more classic perimenopause and menopause symptoms include debilitating hot flashes and night sweats as well as a general loss of motivation and libido. Depression often sets in due to decreased hormones and a loss of quality of life.

One of the long-term issues that can arise with hormone imbalances is that women are told that there is nothing they can do about it—that it is a normal part of aging. Women think they must live with stress, pain, and an inability to sleep, and they often feel the need to medicate themselves (or self-medicate) to manage these issues.

To top it all off, we are now getting exposed to toxic environmental estrogens called xenoestrogens, which are an estrogen imposter that causes chaos in our bodies. These are man-made hormones used as stabilizing agents in beauty care products, household items, cleaning supplies, food storage items, and more. It is estimated that by the time the average woman has completed her morning routine and leaves the house for the day, she has been exposed to more than 126 different chemicals through an average of thirteen different products. Of those numerous chemicals, many are xenoestrogens.

I discovered something very interesting when I was doing my Ph.D. dissertation. I learned that there are women in other cultures, such as the Mayan Indian culture, that do not have any struggles with hormone issues in perimenopause. They do not even have words for "hot flashes" or "night sweats" in their language. There is a natural cessation of the period that happens with the females of these civilizations, but there is nothing negative associated with these changes. As a woman ages, her periods stop, and they have a ceremony where she is celebrated as a wise elder of the village.

In contrast, in more developed nations, menopause is medicalized as if it is a disease. There is much negative stigma surrounding menopause, and women tend to suffer in silence. When comparing our lifestyle to that of the Mayan Indians, we realize that we are not living indigenously as we are intended to live. We are being exposed to many hormone-disrupting foods, chemicals, and habits, and we have poor self-care overall. Our lifestyle is fast-paced, stressful, and rarely harmonious.

Our food has changed more in the past fifty years than it has in the past thousand years. The broccoli we eat is not the same broccoli that our grandparents ate. Fruits and vegetables today are grown in nutrient-depleted soil, densely sprayed with pesticides and often genetically modified, rendering them unrecognizable in some cases. The same thing is true with our bread—our wheat is genetically modified, cross-hybridized, and laden with chemicals and pesticides. The Mayan Indians, for example, are not getting exposed to these chemicals as they are living as close as possible to how their ancestors did. They respect their heritage and carry it forward throughout the generations. This allows them to live a much healthier lifestyle on all levels, and as a result, they have no reported issues with perimenopause or menopause.

Although menopause is a normal part of aging in our lives, the symptoms that are frequently associated with it do not have to be accepted as normal. These symptoms are often treated with pharmaceutical medications called (synthetic) hormone replacement therapy (HRT) that can have harmful side effects. However, many medical doctors are becoming more reluctant to prescribe hormone replacement therapy because of the 2002 study by the Women's Health Initiative that showed it could have potentially damaging effects. This reluctance has led medical doctors to prescribe symptomatic treatment for hormone issues such as anti-depressants, birth control pills, sleeping pills, and hormone secreting IUD's, none of which address the root cause of the issues.

Hormones naturally fluctuate throughout the month, but they can also fluctuate unnaturally in response to lifestyle factors such as poor nutrition, liver toxicity, excess stress, and not getting enough sleep. Fortunately, there are some simple steps that can be taken to balance your hormones!

The main female sex hormones are estrogen, progesterone, and—to a much lesser extent—testosterone. When these hormones become unbalanced, there is often a ripple effect that causes other hormones to go out of balance as well.

The key to healthy and balanced sex hormones is to support the whole body, including the ovaries, adrenals, and thyroid. The adrenal glands are the most common starting point, as they often prove to be the most beneficial to supporting the other hormones.

There are many different types of effective natural therapies that can be used to treat and reverse the underlying causes of hormone imbalances. There are seven key areas to address when attempting to balance your hormones: gut health, liver function, stress reduction, adrenal health, thyroid function, diet, and exercise.

The focus in my practice is to discover which hormones are out of balance and causing the issues you are facing. The main hormones that commonly come into play as a woman approaches and enters menopause are the adrenal hormones (cortisol and DHEA), the thyroid hormones (TSH, free T4, free T3, and the thyroid antibodies), TPO, estrogen, progesterone, testosterone, and insulin. Whether a woman has a thyroid issue, adrenal dysfunction, estrogen dominance, or insulin resistance, I design a customized natural healing protocol to bring the hormones back into balance.

In my practice, I seek out to find the specific hormonal story that is unique to each patient. During an initial appointment with me, we spend over an hour going over your current medical situation as well as past medical health, nutrition, lifestyle, stress, sleep, and so much more. This appointment is the first step in healing. Often women feel so much better after this first appointment because they are finally able to talk about how they are feeling and have someone listen to them. They leave feeling hopeful, which is exactly my mission—to instill hope!

Next, I request comprehensive hormone testing to be done through a combination of blood and saliva samples, which will give me a complete and detailed reading on all of your hormones. Using these results as a guide, I will administer natural remedies such as herbal medicine, supplements, and nutrient therapy. Often, I will also recommend bioidentical hormones to quickly replace deficiencies and resolve symptoms. Bioidentical hormones are natural and are the exact same hormone molecule as what is in a woman's body—this makes them less risky than synthetic hormone replacements.

Nutrition and lifestyle changes are the foundations of my treatment plans. The body relies on having the proper nutrients to produce the hormones that are needed to sustain balance. Consuming a whole food diet that is free from processed foods and excess sugar, and that reduces reliance on caffeine and alcohol, is a crucial step in the healing process. Often in my practice, I will start with a body re-set detoxification program to rid the system of excess toxins; this enables the elimination organs to flush out harmful xenoestrogen buildup. Once the body has been detoxified, we establish a sustainable nutrition plan to continue your healing journey.

There are some simple lifestyle changes that I often recommend as well. Stress identification and management is the most important aspect to achieving balance and maintaining the health of the adrenal glands. This can be achieved by eliminating unnecessary stressors and establishing healthy boundaries—be it with family, work demands, and even self-imposed stress. Sleep is also foundational, and healthy changes often need to be made to ensure you are experiencing adequate and restorative sleep patterns.

The key to finding a successful treatment plan that is going to be effective for you is to find and naturally treat the underlying cause, make the necessary lifestyle and nutritional changes, and live a life that is filled with balance, peace and joy!

Case Study: Andrea

Andrea had been struggling with some hormonal issues for a few years before coming to see me. She had always been healthy and happy until she entered perimenopause. She began noticing these issues around the age of forty-eight, although she brushed them off at first. She thought she was tired because she had been working more. She assumed her mood swings were just due to the extra stress she was under. The weight she had gained was surely because she had not been able to exercise as much as before; her life was just too busy to fit it in. She felt like she was on autopilot, and that one day just turned into the next without much difference.

By the age of fifty-one, she was right on the cusp of entering menopause and began experiencing horrendous cycles that greatly interfered with her life. Her periods were so heavy that there were some days that she was afraid to leave the house!

Andrea did not feel like herself. She had become very depressed and irritable, and she had gained nearly twenty pounds. She wanted to sleep all day and had a hard time dragging herself into work. Night sweats were now regularly interfering with her sleep, and she was having a very hard time concentrating and focusing at work. She had lost her motivation to exercise, or to even socialize that much. She started isolating herself, which was very unusual for her as she used to enjoy weekly outings with friends and family. She was drinking two to three glasses of wine every day for stress relief, almost like a medication. Then, at night, she would feel depressed and turn to sugar to make herself feel better. In the morning, she was so exhausted that she was abusing caffeine. She couldn't figure out what was happening; this was nothing she had ever experienced before, and none of it made any sense.

In our first appointment, Andrea was flooded with emotion as she described how she had been feeling over the past few years. She had come to realize that something must be wrong, because this wasn't like her! She had gone to her family doctor, and out of concern her doctor offered to prescribe her anti-depressants, but she knew that was not the answer.

We began by testing her hormones and, sure enough, they were dramatically out of balance. Andrea's adrenal glands were functioning at a very low level and her thyroid was sluggish. Her family doctor had tested her thyroid previously and it was normal by the standard means of testing, but the detailed testing that I had done showed that

Andrea's free T3 was low. This accounts for why she had gained so much weight, and for some of the fatigue. The testing also revealed that her progesterone was very low compared to her estrogen, which only magnified her menopause symptoms.

I put her on a hormone-balancing regime that included bioidentical hormones, natural thyroid replacement support, adrenal support, and some estrogen and progesterone balancing herbs, combined with additional nutritional and lifestyle changes. Once she began to feel better through the hormone therapies, she was able to address her nutrition and lifestyle. We examined her stress levels and eliminated all the unnecessary things in her life that were causing her so much stress.

This process was so empowering for her that it became easy for her to re-create her life into a version that she could truly enjoy. Within a couple of months, she had experienced a complete turnaround—she was sleeping better, she had sustained energy throughout the day, her moods were balanced, and she could handle stress so much better than before. Over time she lost twenty-two pounds and is now at her ideal weight. She is consistently exercising three times a week and now feels better than she ever has!

Hayley Stobbs, Registered Acupuncturist

I am a registered acupuncturist and nutritional consultant based in Victoria, British Columbia. I work primarily with women, and I also treat individuals recovering from addictions with acupuncture detox.

I am drawn to women's health because modern-day women live a very busy, hectic lifestyle—one that often lacks adequate self-care. Too many women are in a state of deficiency and depletion, exhausted all the time, tired-yet-wired and not motivated to do the things they love. My mission is to raise awareness for self-care through acupuncture, dietary changes, and lifestyle guidance.

Although some of my patients are proactive with their health, the majority of women who arrive at my practice do so after having "hit the wall." This means they are either at a point of complete exhaustion and have finally decided to make their health a priority, or they have unsuccessfully tried other things to reduce or eliminate their unpleasant experiences, such as hot flashes, and someone suggested acupuncture to them.

Acupuncture is a gentle, natural, and effective option for women to deal with symptoms associated with hormone fluctuations during perimenopause and menopause. It doesn't have any adverse side effects, unlike medications, and it is often covered by extended medical coverage.

Perimenopause and menopause are discussed a lot in our training because acupuncture is a modality that is effective and sought after by so many women. It has been shown to reduce hot flashes, anxiety, and mood swings and correct hormonal imbalances. It has health benefits for everyone and may be a good option for any woman who can't use, or chooses not to use, hormone therapy. Women who are bothered by hot flashes and night sweats may want to try acupuncture as it's a relatively low-cost, low-risk treatment.

For women who have "hit the wall," acupuncture balances the yin and yang in the body. Yin and yang are relative terms in Traditional Chinese Medicine, where yin describes the state of being and yang is the state of doing. Yin is nourishing and restful, while yang is about activity. By balancing our nourishment with our activity, we can create a state of hormone balance, both before and after menopause.

Health is defined by yin and yang harmoniously interacting in a dynamic and constantly changing balance. Female sex hormones are predominantly yin; they are consumed by stress hormones, which are yang. If we can focus on regulating (or balancing) the stress hormone cortisol, this will help to take care of estrogen and progesterone balance as well.

Traditional Chinese Medicine views perimenopause and menopause as a natural occurrence. We expend yin by working, stressing, grieving, giving birth, and taking care of others. This means that by the time a woman reaches the perimenopause phase of life, her body may not be as efficient at balancing her natural rhythms of cooling and calming and she may be more irritated, hot, or anxious. She may be struggling to sleep or generally feeling out of balance and not quite herself.

Acupuncture is believed to reduce hot flashes by prompting blood flow and triggering the production of stress- and mood-regulating hormones. As with all treatments, it could also be possible that the placebo effect influences the results of acupuncture; if you believe something will be effective in helping you, there is at least a 30% chance that it will.

Acupuncture does not treat any two people alike. Your acupuncturist will take your medical and emotional history and put together a treatment protocol designed to address your particular symptoms and experiences.

We are trained to insert needles for optimal blood and energy flow, and it doesn't hurt. In fact, most patients are very surprised by the relaxing, meditative effects acupuncture can have.

We typically recommend regular treatments, as the effects are cumulative; this may mean treatments one to two times per week if you are in an acute state of stress. Every treatment plan is individualized, but you can expect to work up to monthly appointments and eventually "tune-up" treatments a few times per year.

I find that acupuncture treatments are most effective when they are incorporated with Traditional Chinese diet therapy too. This includes eliminating excess sugar, caffeine, and processed foods. Yin-nourishing foods include dark berries, fruits, vegetables, and whole foods.

Acupuncturists are trained to work as part of your health team. Expect them to ask you about what other health care practitioners you are working with, such as a naturopathic doctor or family doctor. If acupuncture doesn't produce results within a defined number of treatments, acupuncturists are obligated to refer their patients to another health care practitioner. We always want to give our patients the confidence that if we can't eliminate or improve symptoms, they can trust us to refer them to someone else, because we truly care about their health outcomes.

Case Study: Gayle

Gayle is fifty-three and works in a high-stress environment as a legal assistant. When I meet her, I quickly realize she doesn't like to talk about her work whatsoever. She is bothered by hot flashes and sleep deprivation. Gayle had a hysterectomy when she was forty-nine; she isn't taking any hormone therapy and indicated that her doctor didn't even discuss with her what life might be like post-operation. A work friend recommended acupuncture to her, and that is how she found me.

My recommendations included acupuncture treatments twice weekly for two weeks because she was in an acute state of stress. My first priority is to see if we can restore Gayle's sleep, but I know hot flash reduction is also important as hot flashes are impacting her ability to do her job and function normally. I learn that Gayle has already started magnesium, lavender oil capsules and apple cider vinegar to help manage her blood sugar.

After a few weeks, Gayle told me her work stress is still there, but her sleep was improving and her hot flashes had all but disappeared. The most surprising part? She was not only enjoying the after-benefits of acupuncture, she was also really enjoying the in-treatment time itself. She told me she was actually scheduling "me time." She had never imagined that something like acupuncture, which involved the insertion of fine needles and took her away from her hectic schedule, would be so relaxing and meditative!

Dr. Meghan van Drimmelen, Doctor of Naturopathic Medicine

I first became interested in women's health during my undergraduate studies, where my favourite courses were hormones and endocrinology. Later, during my naturopathic doctor internship, I had the opportunity to work with women, and I was completely fascinated. The ability to inform, educate, and team up with a woman to achieve results was truly empowering for me as a health care professional, and I saw that same empowerment unfold as I saw more and more women at all stages of their reproductive lives. That's when I decided to focus my practice on women's health.

There is a lot that can be achieved via naturopathic medicine—lots of education, lots of available options, and lots of information, all leading to empowerment. I see my patients as travellers, and I am the guide for their own unique journeys.

I talk about empowerment, yet for many women in perimenopause or the very early stages of perimenopause, they initially don't feel very empowered at all! In fact, often they show up in my office unsure why they are feeling the way they are feeling, both physically and emotionally. Some women do a lot of research before coming to meet with me, but many of them end up confused because so much misinformation stems from definitions. Women may be aware that menopause means going twelve months without a period. Sometimes they are aware of the definition of perimenopause, and often times they are also confused by its definition—especially if they have been told it isn't menopause when you still have a period. And yes, that *is* true. It's not menopause when you still have a period, or when your period becomes irregular or heavier—that's perimenopause!

My job as a naturopathic doctor is to connect the dots, provide education and information, and—if the patient's hormones are out of balance—to offer recommendations that will restore their quality of life.

The following is a very common example of a patient in my practice who is trying to navigate her perimenopause journey. Perhaps you can relate, or have a girlfriend or sister with a similar story.

Kate is forty-three. She is feeling overwhelmed and hasn't been sleeping well for the first time in her life—with the exception of when she had her babies. It's frustrating. Her periods have gotten heavier, which is a huge drag and very inconvenient, and she is becoming fed up with it! She always seems to be tired. The fact she has always been healthy until now, coupled with the uncertainty of what is happening to her, is causing her great concern.

When I see women like Kate, I can usually tell right away what they are going through. I am often introduced to women who have already tried very hard to push through what they are experiencing. They want to be proactive with their health, and they are attempting to juggle that task along with a full-time job, kids, a hefty to-do list, and sometimes months or even years of putting themselves on the back burner. Some patients will have already tried over-the-counter remedies such as melatonin. In other cases, the patient's family doctor may have offered birth control pills, which they aren't interested in taking. About half of my first-time patients have looked at and experimented with other options, like those mentioned above, and the other half are landing in my office at the end of their ropes and seeking support.

Naturopathic medicine is in the sphere of complimentary

or integrative medicine; this means that it is complimentary to conventional medical treatments. Doctors of naturopathic medicine are trained to know if a natural remedy is safe and effective to use with the medicine the individual is already taking. We integrate natural and conventional therapies, and we work with the whole health care team. We are trained to perform a thorough intake (medical history), we can order laboratory testing, and we provide physical exams such as Pap tests.

Naturopaths value a holistic approach. We look at the person's body as a whole; this includes physical, mental, emotional, socio-economic, and environmental factors. We try to find the root cause of your symptoms and treat that as a condition, as opposed to providing something that might be more of a band-aid rather than a solution.

Our treatments involve developing a patient-centred, individualized treatment plan. Our main recommendations will always include diet and lifestyle changes along with a personalized action plan that could include nutritional or herbal medicine, acupuncture, intravenous nutrient therapies, and homeopathy. In British Columbia, naturopathic physicians also have prescribing rights for conventional prescriptions and bioidentical hormone therapy, although these rights vary by region.

During an initial naturopathic appointment, we begin with a comprehensive intake form that asks about past health history, family history, any chronic conditions, allergies, lifestyle factors (how you eat, move, sleep, how much water you drink, how much alcohol you drink), any surgeries, any medications and supplements you're taking, your digestion patterns, and your skin health. Once we have this information, we can delve into your main health concerns and discuss your health goals. Patients are encouraged to bring their most recent blood work with them as it is very helpful, and from there we can decide if any other tests are required. The first appointment is always very thorough, and patients tend to appreciate the comprehensive and investigative conversation.

You can also expect a focused physical exam, including taking your blood pressure, palpating the thyroid gland if you are experiencing fatigue, performing an abdominal exam if you have digestive issues, and taking a close look at your skin.

By the conclusion of the appointment, patients can expect to receive information explaining how their symptoms correspond—I call this part "connecting the dots." Sometimes I will send patients home with handouts, lifestyle coaching with diet and nutrition suggestions, and—if required—a requisition for laboratory work.

In the case of women in perimenopause, I like to use a checklist called the Hormone Balance Inventory Tracker (see page 37) that explains some of the main hormones and the functions they are responsible for. It also uses a scale to track the degree to which the woman is experiencing various symptoms. For example, difficulty concentrating or remembering things could indicate a decrease in estrogen or progesterone, and it could also be related to poor thyroid function. I ask the patient to rate this challenge, where "0" means they are non-existent and "20" means there are extreme difficulties. This inventory is used over the course of our time together and it is very helpful for educating how certain experiences correspond to certain hormonal shifts. It also helps to create a picture of how the patient is feeling over time.

My goal for treating any woman in perimenopause is to help her understand the reasons why she is feeling the way she is feeling so she can play a key role in her treatment decisions; one where she feels empowered and optimistic that the course of action we have decided on will work for her. As a doctor, I can suggest my patients eat more green, leafy vegetables, but if the patient doesn't like green vegetables or doesn't know how to prepare them, it's likely not going to work for them. However, if we spend time trying to figure out what *will* work and find a viable solution, such as including greens in a morning fruit smoothie, the patient is much more likely to stick with this recommendation.

One common misconception is that naturopaths are going to automatically prescribe hormone therapy. This is untrue. The type of treatment recommended depends on many factors including patient preference, severity of symptoms, and past medical history and risk factors. In many cases, we take a step-by-step protocol where diet and lifestyle, and natural remedies are recommended first. If that doesn't restore quality of life for the patient, we prescribe bioidentical hormone therapy.

The question I likely get asked the most is: "Are hormones safe?" The short answer is that it depends on the individual. The long answer is yes, so long as age, risk factors, type of hormone, and route of delivery are considered. Hormone therapy is very individualized, and a good clinician should be able to prescribe the best protocol for you and monitor the results.

If you visit a naturopath as part of your perimenopause journey, we always discuss education around hormones and clear up any confusion about the types of hormone therapy. We thoroughly outline the benefits and the risks and talk about proper dosage. If hormone therapy looks like a good course of action, we will discuss a strategy that includes dosage, best route of administration, how often we intend to monitor, and a probable exit strategy. Five years or less used to be the rule of thumb for hormone therapy duration, but now it is recommended that a solution be customized to the individual. The exit strategy will be determined using all the considerations taken when we initially prescribed: her age (is she under sixty?), risk factors, how many years it has been since she reached menopause (has it been ten years or less?), and the severity of symptoms.

When it comes to inviting a naturopathic doctor onto your health care team, people are often curious about how frequently they will need to schedule appointments. As a general rule, for a woman in perimenopause, the second appointment is made for within two to four weeks from the initial visit, and then another four weeks after that. If she is feeling awesome, we book a follow-up in three to four months. In a typical scenario, this works out to approximately four to six appointments in a year.

When anyone is considering seeing a naturopath for the first time, I try to manage their expectations around outcomes. For women navigating hormonal changes, they can expect to feel validated and relieved that they do not have to push through a challenging time with no support. Many of my patients talk about what a huge relief it is when we tell them that everything is going to be okay. Most patients report improved quality of life, improved moods, less stress, fewer hot flashes, and more menstrual regularity as treatment progresses. We also expect our efforts in proactively managing a woman's midlife health to result in improved heart health, bone health, and brain health in the future.

New patients are typically curious about how naturopathic doctors collaborate with family doctors. Within our scope of practice, there are certain things we have to refer out for. For example, we cannot offer certain diagnostic tests like ultrasounds or refer to specialists, so if that is required I will communicate directly with the patient's family doctor. Even if we don't have to refer out, though, I always underscore how important it is for the patient to communicate with her family physician.

I think there is sometimes a myth that naturopathic doctors and medical doctors don't like each other or don't like to work together, making the patient feel timid about telling their family doctor they have other health professionals on their team, not wanting to insult or upset their primary care provider. In my experience, this couldn't be further from the truth; there is mutual respect for both professions, and for any good doctor, the patient's health is the number one priority.

It's impossible for one profession to be able to do everything. Your family doctor might have more training and experience in one area, and I might have more expertise in another. I encourage all my patients to discuss openly and confidently how they are managing their health with all members of their health team. You don't want to walk into your GP's office and simply present a letter from your naturopath; instead, explain how you are and how you have been feeling, then explain you have added a naturopathic doctor to your health team and what he/she has recommended. You should also talk about what you would like to explore, what tests you are interested in pursuing and why you think they will be valuable, and request collaboration. As a naturopath, we don't believe in telling another doctor what to do. We believe two heads are better than one, and we like to work together to fill any gaps.

I find a lot of my work with women who are trying to be proactive with their health in perimenopause comes down to debunking a few myths. I know that perimenopause is not yet very well researched, but there is quite a lot we do know and it's important that more and more women are informed about what to expect. For example, one of the least known parts of perimenopause is what the beginning stages of this life phase entails. Generally speaking, women do not know what signs to be aware of, or what a hormone shift looks like or feels like. Our society has done women a disservice by portraying all women in perimenopause and menopause as having hot flashes. While those are common, the less known and talked about experiences include changes in menstruation, more pronounced PMS, and changes to mood and to sleep patterns. It's important for more conversations around these changes to happen so women know that it's not all in their heads, and that they are not alone.

If I had the chance to tell every thirty-five-year-old woman on the planet four things, it would be to get informed, to listen to your body, to connect with other women, and to keep talking. Not everyone needs external support for their perimenopause-to-menopause journey. However, I invite you to be mindful about your health and start talking about it as soon as you notice changes. Try to incorporate things into your life that you love; this impacts your cortisol, which will then impact other hormones. Be aware of what you put in your body. Eat regularly and be mindful of the quality of food you are eating. Consider a Mediterranean-style diet, or a lower carbohydrate Mediterranean diet, as this helps with cortisol and insulin levels. Also, include movement in your life. Exercise. Walk on your break or after dinner each night. Find something you love to do. We all sit a lot during the day, so it's important to find opportunities to get moving.

What I'd really like to do is write every woman a permission slip that reads, "Not quite feeling like yourself? It's okay to reach out for help!"

Case Study: Elizabeth

When I meet Elizabeth, she is forty-one and her primary concerns include heavy periods, more pronounced PMS, fatigue, difficulty sleeping, stress and anxiety, and low libido.

As usual, I perform a comprehensive medical intake, order bloodwork, and opt for salivary hormone testing. In the earlier stages of perimenopause, I typically go with salivary hormone testing because we tend to get more information from saliva than urine or blood, the reference ranges are a bit more fine-tuned, and we have the opportunity to highlight more health conditions, even if they are at sub-optimal levels. Saliva tests also calculate the estrogen-to-progesterone ratio and cortisol levels. For her blood work, I am looking at her vitamin B12 and iron levels, her thyroid profile, and a marker for hemoglobin A1C (blood sugar).

What we learned was that Elizabeth's iron was low, while her blood sugar and her vitamin B12 levels were fine. Her thyroid profile was not too bad, but her cortisol was low during the day and spiking at night—which is the opposite of what is should be.

Her estrogen, progesterone, and testosterone were all within range. However, her progesterone-to-estogen ratio was low, which is common in perimenopause and is usually responsible for heavier periods and more severe PMS.

My recommendations included taking an iron supplement and including more iron-rich foods in her diet. I also performed lifestyle counselling for cortisol management. This includes carving out more time for herself, eating regularly, following a Mediterranean diet, moving more, and ensuring she incorporates the things she loves and is passionate about into her life.

To improve her progesterone-to-estrogen ratio, I recommended cyclical progesterone (oral, before bed) on the days when she gets her period. This is used to slow down the menstrual cycle and will help with sleep. For her adrenal function, we talk about lifestyle tweaks, exercise, and herbs to improve cortisol levels and help the body cope with stress. These include rhodila, ginseng (which you take in the morning) and magnolia bark (which you take at night). For her heavy periods, I also recommend a tincture to take during her period that contains cinnamon essential oil, which helps to curb the heavy bleeding.

Since her thyroid was borderline, I chose not to treat this right away. This can be caused by adrenal fatigue, which she has, so if we opt to treat the adrenals first, it may not be necessary to treat the thyroid.

Case Study: Jayne

Jayne is fifty-three, and she is post-menopausal. It's been a year and a half since her last period, and she didn't seek any support during perimenopause. This is common with many women—they often don't seek help until the hot flashes get really bad and significantly impact their quality of life, and then they are really motivated to find solutions.

Jayne is experiencing ten to twelve hot flashes during the day, and she is only getting two to three hours of sleep per night. Overall, she is not feeling well, either mentally or physically.

She has vaginal dryness and pain with intercourse. Unsurprisingly, her libido is also low.

Jayne describes her thinking as "foggier than it used to be," and she is experiencing more stress and anxiety than normal. She says her energy level is low, and she knows that her issues with sleeping are likely contributing to her general feeling of not being at the top of her game.

Together, we decide to look at her four-point cortisol and test her estrogen, progesterone, and testosterone levels, along with her thyroid, iron, blood sugar, vitamin B12, and cholesterol.

We learn from Jayne's blood work that her iron levels are okay, as are her vitamin B12 and thyroid function. Her blood sugar and cholesterol levels are borderline. Her estrogen and progesterone levels are low, and her testosterone level is low to normal. Her cortisol doesn't look too bad—it's within the reference range, but on the low side of normal.

To help Jayne improve her quality of life, I gave her information around diet for management of her cholesterol and blood sugar. I go over the benefits of a Mediterranean diet with a lower carbohydrate option. I suggest eliminating refined carbohydrates and give her a handout that explains her options. We discuss wine, and my suggestion is that limiting wine is always a good idea. However, if Jayne is going to have wine, I advise that it is better to have one glass per day rather than saving it all up for the weekend. I also recommend more exercise and regular movement to offset Jayne's mostly sedentary lifestyle and recent weight gain.

To address her foggy thinking, we introduce an omega-3 fatty acid. We often see good changes with lifestyle tweaks alone; however, omega-3 has so many other benefits, including managing things like anxiety and inability to concentrate, that I still choose to recommend it.

For cortisol management, I offer Jayne a choice of either lifestyle tweaks and a herbal remedy, or lifestyle tweaks and IV nutrient therapy. Herbal remedies include rhodiola, ginseng, licorice root, and withania, which she would take daily for three to six months. IV nutrient therapy is another option that would include receiving weekly treatments for four to six weeks.

We discuss her options for low estrogen and progesterone. Because Jayne is a healthy, symptomatic woman in her early fifties with no apparent health history or health risks for breast cancer, heart disease, or blood clotting, we talk about bioidentical hormone therapy and decide to pursue it. I prescribe Bi-est, which is a bioidentical estrogen cream containing estradiol and estriol, and we combine this with an oral micronized progesterone to take before bed and prescribed to address Jayne's hot flashes, vaginal dryness and to help with sleep.

Kim Vopni, Pelvic Health Expert a.k.a. "The Vagina Coach"

I was strongly influenced by a video in grade six that showed childbirth as a bit of a horror show. It scared the heck out of me, and I made a very conscious decision at age eleven to never have children.

At the same time, I knew this was something my own mother had done. And my grandmothers. And my aunts. I saw all these women around me who had had children, and they had clearly survived. So, I became curious. It was both a fascination and a fear.

Fortunately, my mom was very open, and I asked her what it was like. She told me about episiotomies and I thought, *Oh my god, they cut your vagina?* I know there are proper anatomical terms, but at the time "cutting the vagina" was how my pre-teen brain processed the situation.

I hung onto that concept as I continued to ask my mom other questions. She told me of her struggles with back pain, a tummy she didn't like, and her bladder challenges. In fact, she had bladder repair surgery when she was in her fifties. By that time, I was older, and as she shared things with me, I was making mental notes and weighing the pros and cons of whether or not I would have children. As a young adult, I was pretty certain I would not have children. I was not interested in being in a body that had chronic challenges or one that potentially prevented me from being as active as I wanted to be.

Then, I witnessed my sister-in-law give birth and everything changed. It was eye-opening and life-changing. It was exactly the opposite of the images I had built up in my mind. And, it was the opposite of the way media portrayed birth. By this time I was married, and within the next year I was pregnant.

I am someone who is naturally curious, and I like to think of myself as my own best health advocate. I try to be proactive, and for this next big life event, I knew I wanted to be as prepared as possible. I asked my midwife questions. I researched a product called the Epi-No, which is a bio feedback device that helps train the pelvic floor for childbirth, and reduces the chance of tearing and the need for an episiotomy. This philosophy just made so much sense to me, and it was still baffling to realize this information was not common knowledge. How could this approach exist, and still be a secret to most women? I became a distributor for the Epi-No, and thus began my journey to becoming a vagina coach.

I am a personal trainer with a specialized focus on techniques to optimize pelvic floor health in pregnancy, motherhood and along the journey through perimenopause to menopause. I educate, speak, and work as a personal trainer. I collaborate with pelvic floor physiotherapists, midwives, doulas, and anyone who supports women around the life changes of pregnancy, motherhood and menopause. This can often include naturopaths, Chinese medicine doctors, urogynaecologists, obstetrician-gynaecologists and pelvic floor physiotherapists.

What is the Pelvic Floor?

The pelvic floor is an essential group of muscles that forms the base of the pelvis, along with ligaments, tendons, a huge blood supply, and lots of different nerves. They attach to the pubic joint, the tail bone and the sits bones (those two boney parts in your butt cheeks).

Continence is maintained by the pelvic floor muscles that influence the sphincters, help us decide if we need to pee, poo, or fart, and if it is okay to do so. The pelvic floor muscles also keep our organs—the uterus, bladder, and rectum—in place.

Pelvic and spinal stability is also a role of the pelvic floor muscles, as the muscles attach to different points on the pelvis and on the base of the spine. This contributes to our ability to manage different pressures and movements throughout our day.

And, finally, our pelvic floor muscles play a key role in sexual satisfaction, and lack thereof.

Both men and women have pelvic floors and require strength in these muscles to ensure core control and vitality in life. For the purpose of this chapter, we are mainly discussing female pelvic health. And, just in case you're wondering, taking care of the pelvic floor is a job for ALL women, not just women who are sexually active or who have had children.

It is shocking to me that so many women have never learned about the functions of, or the importance of, pelvic health—for both proactive and restorative reasons. Even women who have had children, or have had corrective surgery, are left in the dark. Even when prescribing medication or surgery, few health care providers are taking the time to educate women on optimal pelvic floor care for life and this needs to change. Women deserve to know and they deserve a collaborative approach. As captains of our own midlife health team, we must own this and seek out as many complimentary therapies as we can to ensure we regain and maintain core confidence.

My children learned about sexual health in grade five and again in grade eight, from an amazing sexual health educator who came to their school. The particular program is very open and uses all the right terms which is essential as we try to normalize conversations around pelvic health. I would love to see the grade eight education expand to include information on pelvic health, Kegels and the importance of proactive care.

All young people should learn about how their body works, things that can interfere with proper function, and when and who to go see if something is not working or doesn't feel right.

So many women are currently suffering in silence because they are ashamed, or embarrassed or because they simply don't know help exists. Stress urinary incontinence (leaking with you laugh, cough, sneeze) is advertised as "light bladder leakage" and women are told that it is "just part of being a woman." It is not part of being a woman, nor is it something women need to live with. Incontinence, prolapse and pain are all signals that the body needs help. Yet, so many women believe that what they are experiencing is "normal" because they have given birth, or because they are older. Imagine if women knew as they began to menstruate how powerful and important pelvic health is and that there is support available if things aren't working as they should. According to the Canadian Health Care Reform, the Canadian health care system is critically outdated when it comes to women's pelvic health. Eighty-three percent of college-educated women do not know about the pelvic floor muscles and the role they play in pregnancy and delivery, and one in three women have pelvic floor dysfunction.

I envision a future where women have access to information that could help them avoid pads, drugs and surgery, and if surgery is needed or chosen, they would know how to prepare for it in a way that would result in a more successful outcome and ensure a successful recovery afterward. You see, surgery fixes the problem, but it does not fix what caused the problem; this means the issues have the potential to persist and repeat. This is why I often hear things like, "Surgery didn't work for me," or "I need to have surgery again."

I'd like to see pelvic floor physiotherapy offered as the first line of defense to assess and treat:

- **Incontinence:** Stress urinary incontinence is when leaking occurs during exertion, such as a laugh or sneeze or jump or run. Urge incontinence occurs when there is a sudden, overwhelming urge to urinate that often results in not making it to the bathroom in time. Mixed incontinence occurs when there is a combination of both.

- **Organ Prolapse:** Prolapse occurs when one or more of the organs (bladder, uterus or rectum) move out of their optimal position and begin to bulge into the vagina. The feeling of prolapse is often described as a feeling of "something is in there" or "something is falling out."
- **Pelvic Pain:** Pain with sex, pubic joint pain and sacroiliac (SI) joint pain are common, especially in pregnancy or after injury such as a car accident.

  Pelvic floor physiotherapy is effective both proactively and restoratively and it is quite likely one of the most underused health resources available to women. It is still very common for women not to know about it, and many physicians do not yet recommend pelvic floor physiotherapy. The medical community does a good job when the solution is pharmaceuticals or surgery, but so often these can be avoided. Unfortunately our current health care system is reactive and treats symptoms rather than taking a proactive approach.

Raising awareness about pelvic health and pelvic floor physiotherapy would play a huge role in preventing so many challenges women face as they age, whether it is from pregnancy, from new experiences in perimenopause and menopause, or from other surgeries or car accidents or movement exercises that aren't ideal for them. I always encourage women to dig deeper and explore beyond what the traditional medical community offers.

I am an advocate for every single woman seeing a pelvic floor physiotherapist—especially in pregnancy. It's the perfect opportunity to make sure the pelvis and surrounding muscles are optimized for delivery. It also helps minimize or pre-empt the aches and pains that are frequently dismissed as "normal" during pregnancy. I'd also like to see women educated about the biomechanics of birth and what they could be doing to prepare for their recovery.

So, to answer the question of when the best time is to see a pelvic floor physiotherapist, the answer ranges from as soon as possible, to when you are pregnant, to today!

Now that you've had your eyes opened to the important role a healthy pelvic floor plays in your health throughout your life, I am hereby passing the baton to you so you can influence others in your circle. You are in a position to influence and word of mouth is very powerful! As women's health advocates, we all share the responsibility of promoting pelvic health to others.

How Much Does It Cost?

Pelvic floor physiotherapy is an investment in your health. Unfortunately, cost can be a barrier for many women.

Typically, pelvic floor physiotherapy fees range from $100-$130 per hour. Here is something to think about: if you experience incontinence, when you choose the pelvic floor physiotherapy route, commit to the work and choose to be proactive with your health, you are likely looking at $200-$400 a year. Compare that to the person who does nothing and spends close to $1500/year for incontinence pads. While pelvic floor physiotherapy is not paid for by medical service plans in Canada, the service is covered by many extended health insurance programs. You may be interested to know that the Government of France pays for postpartum pelvic floor physiotherapy, because that is the opportune time to support healing and set the path for pelvic health for life. Imagine what a load that would take off of the health care system, including days missed from work. Wouldn't it be amazing if the government stepped up and paid for physiotherapy sessions for all women but especially for pregnant and postpartum women? This would ultimately set women up with health and confidence throughout all their life phases.

Common Questions and Comments:

"I really have to come and see you."

I hear this all the time from women who are experiencing challenges, ask me how I can help, tell me that they really need to make an appointment...and then they don't because "they don't have the time."

I understand how busy life is. However, I invite you to think about this: Do you have time for six to eight weeks of post-operation recovery? Do you have time to be off work, not able to earn your income or do the things that bring you joy? Do you have time to manage the frequent trips to the bathroom?

If you are experiencing symptoms, it is your body asking for help. A few one-hour appointments can be life changing and potentially mean you don't need pads, drugs or surgery. Choose to take back control. It will significantly improve so many aspects of your life.

"Should I see you, or should I see a pelvic floor physiotherapist?"

Ideally, both. Pelvic floor physiotherapists are physiotherapists who have additional training in the pelvic floor. They will use gloved fingers to assess the external genitalia and internal structures, looking for abnormalities in skin and tissue. They insert their fingers into the vagina to assess tone, the position of the organs, and the ability of the muscles to contract and relax in a balanced way. They address any pain or discomfort and help you work to reduce or eliminate that stimulus. You will typically see a physiotherapist for a few sessions, learn how to do a Kegel, and be prescribed some specific retraining exercises.

After seeing a pelvic floor physiotherapist, you will feel better, your symptoms will be reduced, and you will want to resume your regular exercise and movement routines. Without knowledge about how to move with awareness and in ways that support pelvic health, women can undo some of the work they accomplish with the physiotherapist. That's where the work I do comes in. It's very important to know how to get moving again without undoing the hard work and progress you have already achieved.

The work I do includes some regular fitness training, plus some specialized techniques including posture awareness and some alignment work (how the body and skeleton is aligned) and hypopressives (a low-pressure exercise technique that couples specific postures with rhythmic breathing). I like to show women how to move and give them increased awareness of what they are actually feeling in their body. I also offer modifications to exercises so they can resume an appropriate level of movement, exercise, and fitness while optimizing their pelvic health for life.

I also assess for diastasis recti (the gap between the two "six-pack" muscles that results in inability to generate and maintain tension in the inner core). This condition is strongly correlated with pelvic floor dysfunction. One hundred percent of women experience diastasis recti during pregnancy. It is completely normal, as this is what makes room for the baby in the growing uterus. What isn't normal is when the distance remains wider than optimal after birth, and the connective tissue that is meant to hold them in place isn't able to generate the tension required for stability. Because the two rectus muscles attach onto the pelvis, it directly influences the pelvis itself and the stability of the pelvic floor.

"Is there anything I can do by myself?"

Yes, there are a number of things you can do on your own to step up your pelvic health!

If leaking is an issue, pay attention to what makes you leak. That's a clear sign that an activity is not appropriate for you—at least not at this time. Try to do it differently, or find a different exercise and then progress back to the one that is currently creating symptoms. Often, exercises that are high impact are the worst culprits, and you may need to switch to lower impact exercises temporarily. I'm not saying the only thing you can do is walk or swim, but know that you have lots of options that can reduce impact and pressure and still give you an effective workout.

I also encourage all my clients to sit less and move more. It's okay to sit, and it's okay to stand, but I suggest you don't do either all day; try to move more often and in a variety of ways. We tend to sit for long periods of time in postures that don't allow our core to work as it should, and as a result, it starts to become stagnant and tight. Then, when you are up and moving around, the pelvic floor can remain stuck and not respond well to everyday things such as laughing, coughing, or sneezing. Practice sitting with a neutral pelvis where your sits bones and vulva are on the surface of your chair rather than the back part of your sits bones and tail bone.

You can learn more by watching some of my videos, which you can find by searching for Kim Vopni, The Vagina Coach on YouTube.

Diet and hydration are also key. You want to adopt a diet that includes adequate fibre and water to ensure there is no straining during bowel movements, as that is damaging to the pelvic floor. Constipation can be a common problem with our busy, stressful lives; it can also be an experience that comes up during hormonal fluctuations in perimenopause.

When leaking occurs, one of the first things women do is start to restrict fluids. This increases constipation! What happens next is the urine becomes more concentrated, making you feel you have to pee more often! So, in trying to prevent one issue, you actually create another one. Note that caffeine can also be an irritant. Take out what is irritating the bladder and replace it with water!

"What should I know about sexual satisfaction?"

Plenty! Even if you have no concerns or symptoms, I highly recommend you go see a pelvic floor physiotherapist every year. You can talk with her about sexual function and learn how to sit and stand in order to enhance sexual health. Sex itself is good for the pelvic floor; sex and orgasms are excellent components of pelvic floor training. Use sex as an opportunity to investigate, research, and connect with your pelvic floor. Use your partner and yourself, or a biofeedback toy, to learn and practice. For example, you can say "Can you feel me hugging you?" or "Can you feel when I am letting go?"

"Why didn't anyone tell me about this before?"

If you're just learning about pelvic health for the first time, you are not alone. Perhaps it is lack of awareness, or perhaps it is because pelvic health is still a taboo topic. For now, women need to take matters into their own hands. The good news is there are more and more pelvic health advocates working to change perceptions in media, the medical community and even conversations with girlfriends and around the water cooler. The more professionals we have talking about pelvic health, the faster change will happen.

The Biggest Myths about Pelvic Health

One of the first myths is that **leaking is normal** after you've had children. Perhaps it happened to your mother or grandmother, and you assume it's a natural part of getting older. It is not. Incontinence pads should be a temporary option. They manage the symptom but do not treat the problem.

Another myth is that **surgery is inevitable** or that it is the best option. Women think it excludes them from having to do "all those exercises," when what they really need to do is commit to lifestyle modifications that will ensure optimal pelvic health for the rest of their lives.

The next myth that comes up is that **constipation is common**. Okay, this one is actually true—constipation is common. We drink less water, consume many more processed foods than we should, and we sit too much. The connection between constipation and pelvic floor health is not well known or understood by the general public. Some women experience a feeling of incomplete elimination, and this can be a symptom of prolapse when the rectum has bulged into the vagina and stool can actually get trapped in there, giving the feeling that a bowel movement is never complete.

Many people believe that **holding your tummy in is good for your core** when actually it leads to constipation. Women in particular—and some men too—will hold their abs in all day, which interferes with digestion and creates constipation and gas. It also puts a lot of pressure downwards on the pelvic floor.

There's also a common belief that **there's nothing wrong with wearing tight clothing**, such as jeans or restrictive shape wear. In reality, clothing that is too tight influences how we move throughout the day; it affects how we walk and bend and creates holding patterns that can lead to constipation and pelvic floor dysfunction.

One myth I can't wait to bust is that **incontinence is synonymous with menopause**. The fluctuation in estrogen that occurs during perimenopause, at menopause and post-menopause contributes to the thinning of the muscles and tissues in the bladder and pelvic floor. This does not mean that incontinence is inevitable. By being proactive with your pelvic health and choosing annual pelvic floor physiotherapy, you can thrive in midlife and beyond without experiencing incontinence.

A final common myth is that workouts must include a minimum of an hour of cardio and thirty minutes of weights and stretching. This kind of thinking is outdated, which is good news for most women. I can't emphasize this enough: simply sitting less and moving more will help. I also recommend women choose shorter cardio sessions that respect the pelvic floor but still get you out of breath and sweating. Elliptical machines, spin classes, hill walking and high intensity interval training with weights are all good options. Ensure resistance training with body weight or dumbbells is part of your weekly fitness to help build and maintain bone density and muscular strength and endurance.

In conclusion, if there was one thing I could say to every thirty-five-plus-year-old woman, is that you need a vagina coach! It's all about feeling empowered and knowing your body—how to move it, how it responds, and what works best for you. Remember:

- The pelvic floor loves to move. Sit less, move more, and move with awareness.
- Incorporate more natural movement into your day—walk, squat, take the stairs.
- Stay hydrated.
- Keep reading, get informed, watch videos, and spread the word, because when you do all these things, you are truly being your own best health advocate!

Case Study: Connie

Connie is forty-eight and has three children ages fifteen, twelve, and eight. Her first was a vaginal delivery with an episiotomy, and she experienced tearing with her second. She was in a back-lying position for all three. She is married but doesn't have a lot of sex, and she doesn't really enjoy it when she does.

Connie is a runner, and her main complaint is that she leaks when she runs. She wears pads while exercising, but other than that she hasn't done too much about it. She has a little bit of back pain, but it is not chronic.

Even though Connie runs all the time and her diet is very good, she still feels "pudgy." She knows she ought to be lifting weights, but she also feels that she doesn't have enough energy to do so.

Her periods are heavy, and she is finding that she has more leaking right before her period (which is a glimpse into what she may face in post-menopause). She has never heard of a pelvic floor physiotherapist before. Connie's comment to me (which I hear a lot) is, "I'm not really sure why I'm here, but my friend told me I should see you."

Because pelvic floor dysfunction is not talked about openly, referrals from girlfriends is often the only way women learn that they are not alone, and that there is help and support available.

During my first assessment with Connie, I notice she has a functional diastasis recti, which means she can generate tension in her abdominal muscles but needs some work in maintaining it. I also find that she has some non-optimal holding/movement patterns and she has difficulty recruiting her pelvic floor without using other muscles to help.

My recommendations for Connie include:

- Stop running or reduce the distance (for the time being).
- Go see a pelvic floor physiotherapist.
- Work on alignment: With every client, I assess their stance and how they hold their body, which is essentially their posture. Alignment is the byproduct of working on better posture.
- Body awareness: I take a before and after photo and point out how she currently stands versus how she should be standing.
- Release work: hamstring and calf lengthening (stretching), pelvic floor release, psoas release (free video available on my website), finding the best cue and teaching the core breath, showing her how to release what is holding her in a non-optimal form, and teaching her how her core and pelvic floor can now work better together

- Core breath work/Kegel demonstration: We go over the definition of a Kegel and how Connie can find her best cue and bring that into the movement. Women often need retraining for how to lift a child or a bag of groceries.
- Hypopressives (low pressure fitness): These are a series of low-pressure postures coupled with a rhythmic breathing pattern and an apnea (breath hold) in order to create a vacuum effect that draws everything up. Over time, when done consistently, hypopressives can be very effective for incontinence and early stage prolapse. While I don't think Connie is experiencing early stage prolapse, prevention is essential.

I invite Connie to go away with this list, do the release work for a couple weeks, and then come back. By the next time I see her, she wants to go back to running. However, before we re-introduce running, my goal is to get her sweating and get her heart rate up by lifting weights. I want to see her work out within a twenty-minute time frame, and to do it with exercises that are safe for her pelvic health. Yes, my goal is always to get more results in less time!

By the third time I see Connie, she is feeling stronger and experiencing less leaking. Three months later, she is leak-free, her back pain is gone, she is feeling less "pudgy," and she is even noticing more definition in her muscles. She walks every day with some hills and stairs instead of running and feels she has more free time now that she has shortened her workouts.

When I ask her if she is pleased with the results, Connie tells me she initially thought I was going to be a trainer who prescribed some crazy ab workout! She is more than pleased with the results she was able to achieve, as well as the education and training she received. Now she has become such an advocate for pelvic health, that she is constantly telling her friends the tips and tricks for a healthy pelvic floor.

Part III

What's Next

What's Next

Too many women are making limited health decisions due to limited access or limited financial resources.

Women thirty-five to sixty-five hold the most influential positions in society and the most consumer buying power. They are literally holding our world up right now. Yet, women's top health concerns are not being adequately addressed. This is what keeps me awake at night. It's 2018 and women are still being told "you're too young for menopause," "if you still have a period, it's not menopause" (in response to hormone fluctuations in perimenopause), and "just have a glass of wine" (in response to vaginal dryness or pain with sex) or "it's just part of being a woman; suck it up."

Seventy-seven percent of women don't know what do when it comes to many of their health questions. Sixty-two percent lack time to research. Thirty-one percent don't trust online information. Thirty-five percent don't trust their physician (Harvard Business Review 2015) and seventy percent of women say they don't have anyone to talk to about perimenopause or menopause (Menopause Chicks, 2016).

It was that last statistic that led to the launch of the Menopause Chicks Private Online Community two years ago. We currently have over six thousand members who are generating between ten and fifteen thousand questions and comments each month. That's a lot of questions about women's health, and we haven't even scratched the surface.

We are not taking care of women. The model is broken and it's time to do something about it.

Navigating perimenopause and menopause is a business. Whole industries have been built around the fact that 100% of women will experience this life phase.

My business, for example, is addressing the gaping hole that exists for women looking for quality education and peer support.

And navigating women's health can also be expensive: building your health care team, buying quality vitamins and supplements, eating good, wholesome food, going to yoga, trying acupuncture, buying a quality bed and going after that quality sleep—all of it ASSUMES you have adequate financial resources and adequate disposable income to spend on your health. All of it ASSUMES you have health insurance- and extended health coverage.

But what if you are a woman who doesn't have access to those things? And, I don't necessarily mean only women living below the poverty line. What if you are someone who simply has to juggle life's priorities without much left over at the end of the month for investing in your health?

Maybe seeing a naturopath or registered acupuncturist would be just the thing to take care of your adrenals and set you up for a healthy perimenopause transition. But you don't have extended health coverage.

Maybe you'd thrive if you could only boost your health with some iron, magnesium, omega 3s and vitamin B, C & D. But you can't possibly afford to look down the vitamin aisle, let alone shop there every month.

What if your doctor recommends you get the HPV vaccine or hormone therapy or other prescription, but it's not covered and it costs $700? Do you get the vaccine or do you put brakes on your car?

What if you are a doctor who also has to deal with making limited recommendations to patients—perhaps you're sitting with a female patient who you know would benefit from counselling, but you also know she doesn't have the financial means?

It's overwhelming, right?

And if such a health injustice was happening to our children or pets, we'd be the first to step up and do something. Sometimes we act like the system is too big to change. I say: we ARE the system.

We might not be able to empower ALL women, but that should not prevent us from empowering SOME; from at least starting to address this mokita.

That's why we are starting a fund for women whose health options are limited due to limited resources. A percentage of sales from our MOKITA events and from this MOKITA book will go toward starting the MOKITA fund. I do not know where this could go or grow...but I do know this:

THIS IS IMPORTANT.

We are months away from sending four humans to Mars and thankfully there is a well-thought-out health plan in place for them while on their journey.

The least we can do is create the same for the women who are holding up our world closer to home.

Thank you for being here, and sharing with your friends.

#empoweredwomenempowerwomen
#empoweredformidlife
www.MOKITALive.com

Thank You

She believed she could, so she did. That was the temporary tattoo I wore at a retreat I hosted in Whistler in 2016.

Except, it should have said: She believed, and suddenly a universe of friends, family and followers rallied around so she could. The journey to these final pages has not been a smooth one, and I am so grateful for all the hills, valleys and learning along the way.

What has been smooth, though, is the outpouring of unconditional encouragement, cooperation and support.

To my co-authors, Liz, Christine, Andrea, Anna, Jen, Regina, Angela, Bob, Bal, Cobi, Hayley, Meghan and Kim: thank you for seeing the vision and saying yes.

To the team at Influence Publishing, Julie, Danielle, Greg, Judith & Lee: look what happens when you do great work! I'm hooked now!

To all the women who show up in the Menopause Chicks Private Online Community: thank you for asking great questions, getting informed and choosing the journey that's right for you!

To the many, many health professionals who continue to be passionate about igniting a new model for women's midlife health: my eternal gratitude.

For making my dreams come true: thank you Don, Ryan, Keira & Baxter. xo

And to YOU, thank you for picking this book up and sharing it with the women you love.

And for your inspiration & guidance:

Sheila Alwell
Jill Angelo
Adera Angelucci
Jann Arden
Safia Barr
Sandra Barnes
Shelagh Begg
Melody Biringer
Tara Bishop
Michelle Blane
Brené Brown
Debbie Brown
Taryn Brumfitt
Sue Buchan
Nancy Chapman
Clara Cohen
Andrea Coutu
Pauline Dantas
Rochelle David
Sharon Davis
Lisa Deputter Allen
Nicklas Erlich
Louisa Flinn
Jane Fonda
Janine Francks
Lynda Gerty
Susan Gibson
Elisabeth Gill
Sara Gottfried
Mona Hamm
Linda Harwood
Bernice Holden
Susan Johannson
Kerri Johannson
Gladys Johannson
Deanna Jones
Colleen Kelly
Brenda Kirk
Tammie Kocher
Inga Kruse
Donna Leeder
Erin Lowe
Dana Lyseng
Jennifer MacMillan
Deb Manders
Teresa Marshall
Kristina Matistic
Ric Mazereeuw
Tracey McCrae
Tara McIntosh
David Merry
Juliette Morton
Barb Mowat
Jennifer Nadel
Noreen Neuman
Christina Newberry
Christiane Northrup
Greg Nosaty
Nancy Owens
Hayley Owens
Karen Panabaker
Sandra Peat
Sylvie Peltier
Jerilynn Prior
Kristy Prouse
Marie Robinson
Sherry Rollings
Debi Rumley
Marla Shapiro
Haydée Skeet
Sarah Smith
Tobin Smith
Sherry Steele
Amy Stewart
Sue Sullivan
Dana Suzukovich
Shannon Svingen-Jones
Mikaela Taylor
Shannon Thomas
Carolyn Trotter
Maria Turnbull
Tracy Uchida
Don Weir
Joyce Weir
Sheila Weir Ward
Katya Wilson
Oprah Winfrey
Leah Zille
Marnie Goldenberg
Brenda Rouse

Resources

I'm thrilled to share the following resources with you as you begin—or continue—to build your own midlife health team.

This section features my distinguished co-authors (in alphabetical order) as well as a selection of health professionals and businesses—all who are passionate about women's health and believe in the mission of Menopause Chicks.

Co-Authors

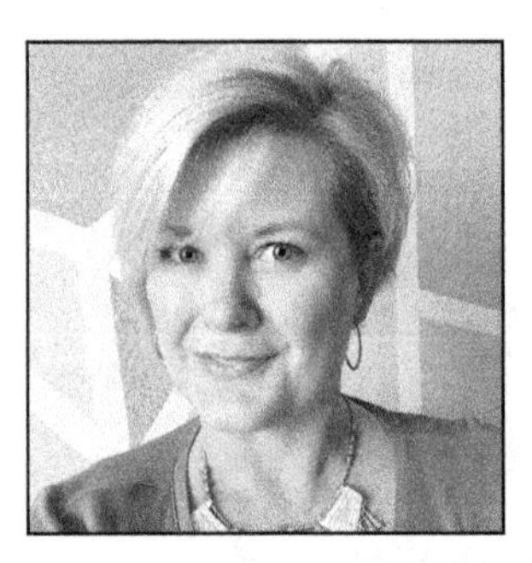

Liz Applegate
Life Coach
ElizabethApplegate.com

Liz is a midlife empowerment coach who enables women to rewrite their next chapter. Her forties included perimenopause, divorce, remarriage, blending families, children flying the nest, an emergency hysterectomy and several career changes. Lack of resources or positive vibrant, voices served as the catalyst for Liz wanting to support other women on similar journeys. Liz hosts a popular podcast at MidlifeSchmidlife.com.

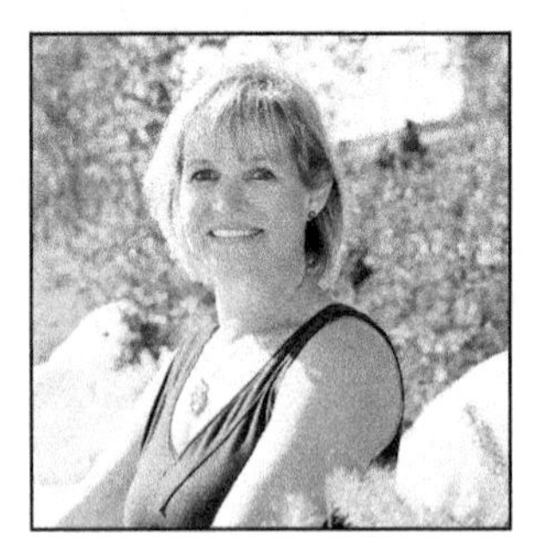

Christine Brain
Integrative Energy Healer
AnahataHypnotherapy.com

Christine is a clairvoyant, certified integrative energy healer and yoga instructor. She combines modalities such as healing touch, craniosacral therapy, guided meditation and Shamanism to treat pain, anxiety, depression, migraines, trauma, abuse and chronic illness, and to support women with their midlife health goals.

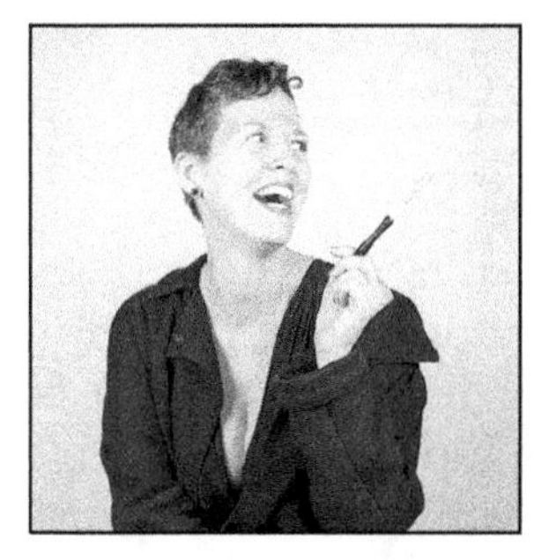

Andrea Dobbs
Women's Health & Cannabis Advocate
VillageBloomery.com

Andrea's mission is to redefine the role cannabis plays in women's health, and to improve access to quality cannabis for all. Andrea's distinguished retail career has focused on buying, merchandising and human resources with forward-thinking retailers like IKEA, The Body Shop and Womyns' Ware Inc. She is the co-founder of The Village Bloomery, an award-winning shop located near Granville Island in Vancouver.

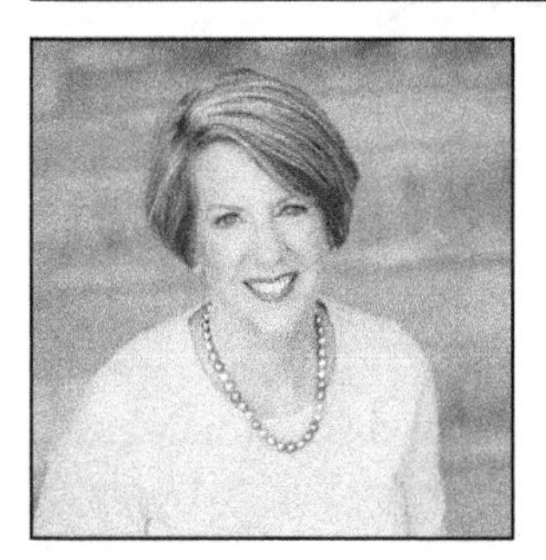

Dr. Anna Garrett
Hormone Balance Expert
DrAnnaGarrett.com

Anna is a hormone balance expert, certified coach and doctor of pharmacy. She works with women in person and around the world who are sick and tired of being sick and tired, and gets their hormones back in balance. Anna is the author of *The Savvy Sister's Guide to Hormone Harmony in Perimenopause.*

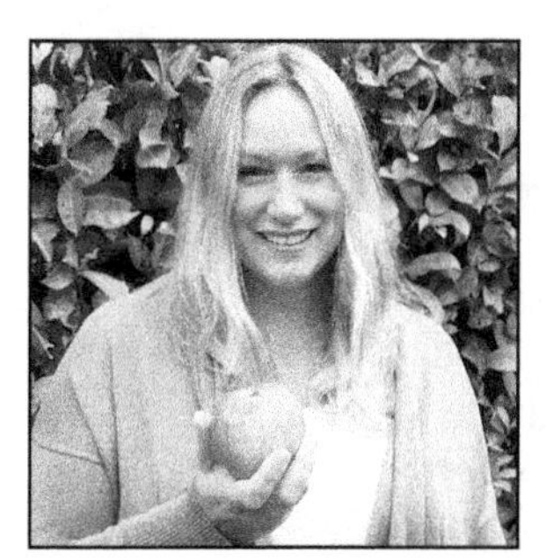

Jennifer Howker, RD
Registered Dietitian
AppleTreeNutrition.ca

Jennifer is a registered dietitian with the College of Dietitians of BC and a member of Dietitians of Canada. She believes the best approach to midlife health is an individualized one that looks at the whole woman. Jennifer's areas of expertise include digestive health, nutrition for optimal mental health, heart health, diabetes management, nutrition for the elderly and nutritional support through perimenopause.

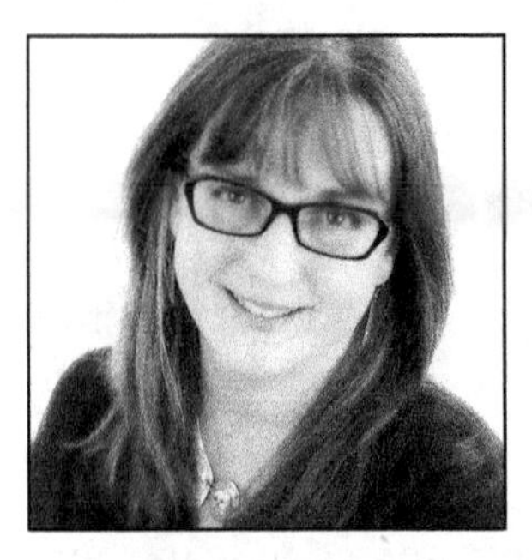

Regina Kaiser
Meditation Teacher & Coach
Veracis.ca

Regina is a certified meditation teacher, yoga instructor, healer, intuitive aromatherapist, and founder of Veracis Meditation, Yoga & Wellness Centre. She integrates knowledge from life experiences with academic studies in natural health and healing, spirituality, meditation and mindful business development. Her teachings are for women looking to live life with awareness and compassion.

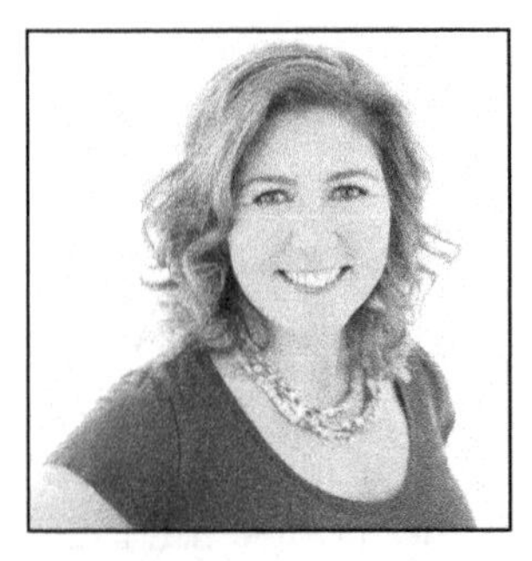

Dr. Angela Macdonald, DC
Chiropractor
PartnersinHealthMR.com

Angela graduated summa cum laude from Western States Chiropractic College in Portland, Oregon. Her clinic, Partners in Health, consists of a multi-disciplinary team committed to helping people "seize the day!" Dr. Macdonald is passionate about posture and loves how Foundation Training can re-wire poor patterns in order to reduce pain, increase strength and reclaim health and vitality.

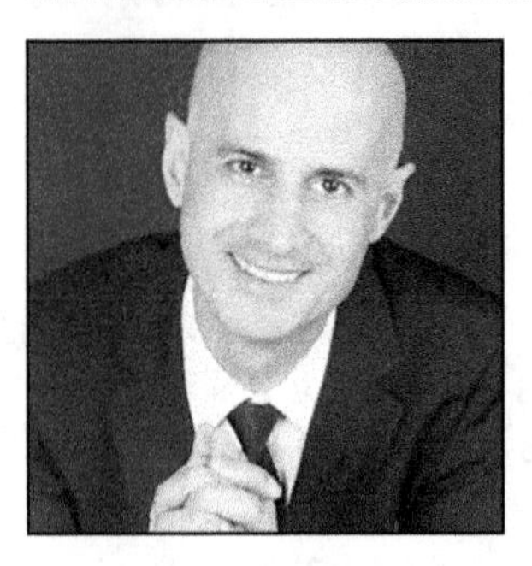

Bob Mehr, B.Sc. (Pharm)
Pharmacist
PurePharmacy.com

Bob is president & CEO of Pure Integrative Pharmacy, which he began, with his wife, Mahtab, from the understanding that the pharmaceutical approach to health and wellness needed a new direction: a focus on promoting vitality and preventative medicine. Bob's vision combined a holistic and integrative health model with traditional pharmacy services and in doing so, he has created a chain of pharmacies like no other.

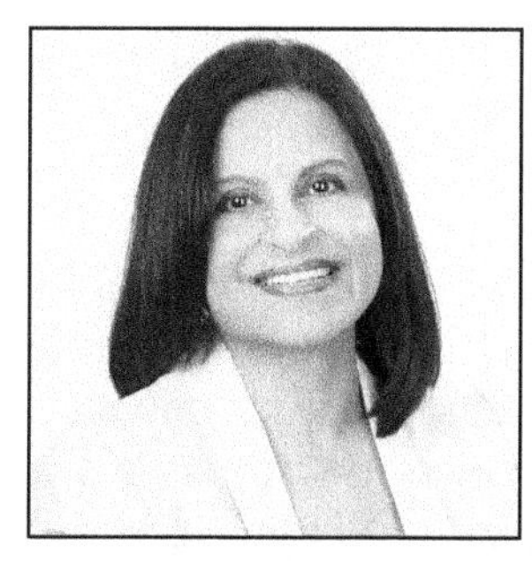

Dr. Bal Pawa, B.Pharm, MD
Integrative Physician
WestCoastWomensClinic.com

Bal is a physician specialist in women's health, pharmacist, certified menopause clinician through the North American Menopause Society and co-founder of the West Coast Women's Clinic for Hormone Health. As a women's health advocate, Dr. Pawa is passionate about evidence-based, integrative medicine, and she inspires future physicians as a clinical instructor at the University of British Columbia's School of Medicine.

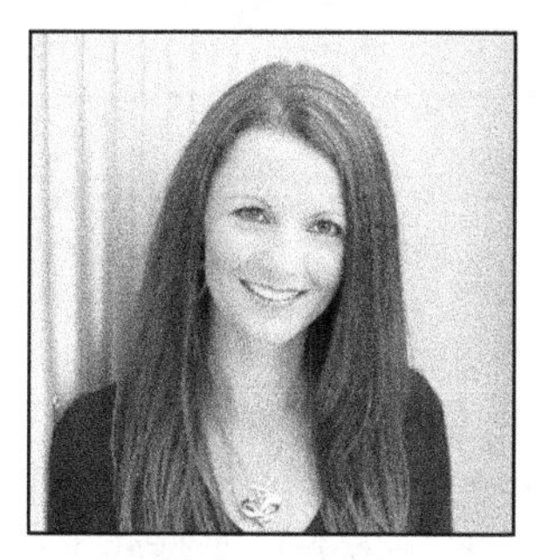

Dr. Cobi Slater, PhD, DNM, CHT, RNCP
Doctor of Natural Medicine
DrCobi.com

Cobi is a board-certified doctor of natural medicine, registered herbal therapist, registered nutritionist and holds a PhD in natural health sciences. She is the founder of Essential Health Natural Wellness Clinic in Maple Ridge, BC and also consults with patients online. Dr. Cobi is an expert in hormonal health, extremely passionate about empowering midlife women, and she is the author or numerous books.

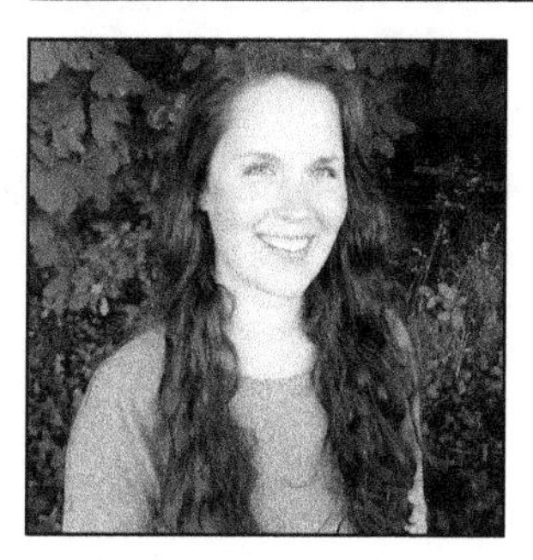

Hayley Stobbs, R.Ac., CNC
Registered Acupuncturist
InnerPassAcu.com

Hayley is a registered acupuncturist and certified nutritional consultant. She supports her patients through menstrual irregularities, fertility and pregnancy, perimenopause and menopause, thyroid and adrenal health, muscle tension, migraines, stress, anxiety, insomnia, allergies and digestive health. Services include acupuncture, Gua sha, cupping, acupressure, moxibustion and nutritional consulting.

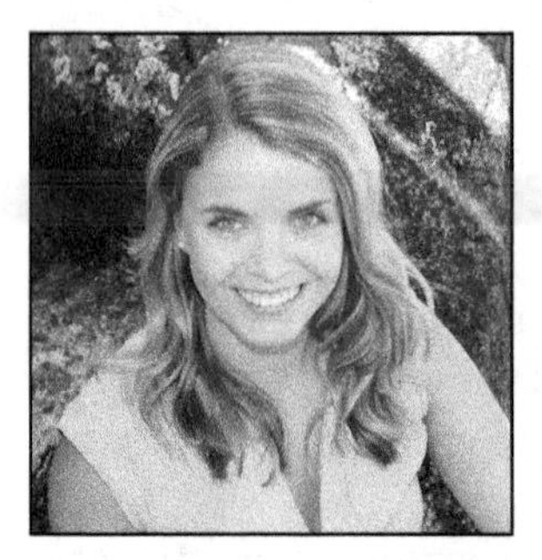

Dr. Meghan van Drimmelen, ND
Doctor of Naturopathic Medicine
JuniperFamilyHealth.com

Meghan is an expert in the field of women's health. Areas of specific interest include hormone balance, perimenopause, menopause, skin and digestive concerns, support for mental health, fatigue and allergies. Dr. van Drimmelen is licensed with the College of Naturopathic Physicians of British Columbia and holds certifications in pharmaceutical prescribing, acupuncture and intravenous nutrient therapy. She has also received advanced training in bioidentical hormone therapy, gynaecology and obstetrics.

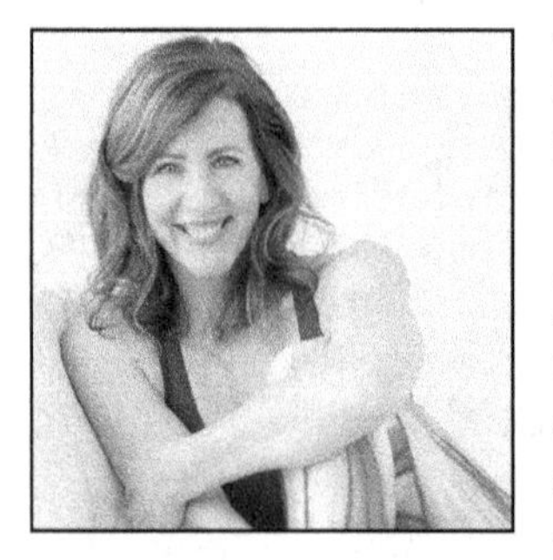

Kim Vopni
Pelvic Health Expert a.k.a The Vagina Coach
VaginaCoach.com

Kim's mission is to help women optimize their pelvic health in pregnancy, motherhood and menopause. She is a restorative exercise specialist, and certified as a personal trainer, pre/post natal fitness consultant, fitness for fertility specialist, pilates instructor and hypopressive method trainer. Women who work with Kim are able to address incontinence issues, reduce/eliminate prolapse symptoms, improve posture, improve and learn how a strong pelvic floor is an essential key to living a life of vitality.

Additional Resources

Kira Cai, ND, Adrian Yeong, ND, Victor Chan, ND
Naturopathic Doctors
SCIMEDICAHealth.com

We asked: What is the one thing you want women to know about perimenopause? **Dr. Kira Cai said:** Every day, I see women in perimenopause, and I am a woman navigating perimenopause myself. I can assure you the symptoms we often hear about do not have to play a significant role in your life. The underlying causes are hormone related and they can be reduced or eliminated with the right information, focus and treatment strategies.

Laureen Card
Transformational Coach
LaureenNowlanCard.ca

We asked: What is the one thing you want women to know about perimenopause? **Laureen said:** Trust yourself! Your body, heart and soul are speaking to you. They will be quiet no more. Listen to your inner wisdom. What you are experiencing is real and there are resources to help you. This is a well-travelled path and you do not need to do this alone.

The Centre for Menstrual Cycle and Ovulation Research (CeMCOR)
Cemcor.ubc.ca

The Centre for Menstrual Cycle and Ovulation Research (CeMCOR) is dedicated to women's health research and interpreting scientific data to empower women as they progress through the natural stages of life. CeMCOR's founder, Dr. Jerilynn Prior, BA, MD, FRCPC, is a professor of endocrinology at the University of British Columbia. She has dedicated her career to studying menstrual cycles, perimenopause, menopause and osteoporosis. CeMCOR's website fields between 3500-7000 page views per day!

Harmonie Eleveld, ND
Naturopathic Doctor
NaturalChoiceMedicalClinic.com

We asked: What is the one thing you want women to know about perimenopause? **Dr. Harmonie said:** I want women to know suffering is not "normal"! Many women wait a long time before seeking help. They assume they have to put up with symptoms affecting their quality of life. It's not true. Hormones affect every area of our body and if you think your experience could be related to hormone fluctuation in perimenopause, you are probably right! There are many treatment options available.

Genneve
Genneve.com

Big life transitions are easier with a team. No one expects you to be the expert at everything or do it all on your own. Perimenopause and menopause are natural transitions that can include both joys and challenges. We are the place for connections with health professionals, healthy products, and forums for conversation with other women who've been where you are.

Kelly Greer, RD
Registered Dietitian
Nutrigal.ca

We asked: What is the one thing you want women to know about perimenopause? **Kelly said:** The emotional shifts during perimenopause can be scary. I want women to know there is no shame in falling apart. I want women to let go of the insane expectations. Do the best you can, rest, ask for help, and remember: it's okay to say f*ck it and go to the beach for the day.

Irene Hogan, B. Pharm. Hons, RPh, NCMP
Menopause Expert
IreneHogan.com

We asked: What is the one thing you want women to know about perimenopause? **Irene said:** I want women to understand perimenopause and menopause are not diseases. As transformational life phases, they are also not for the faint of heart! With the right tools and resources, your symptoms can be managed and you can live your life with passion and vitality. Your body was not meant to break during this stage of life. You deserve to thrive through perimenopause, menopause and beyond!

Kristy Prouse, MD, FRCSC (Ob.Gyn)
The Institute for Hormonal Health
HormonalHealth.ca

Dr. Kristy Prouse is the medical director at The Institute for Hormonal Health (IHH), specializing in the treatment of health issues that are hormonal in origin. The focus is on the whole patient to get to the root of the problem. With an unparalleled team of medical professionals, IHH combines the evidence-based science of both western medicine and naturopathic medicine with nutritional support. Many people don't realize bladder leakage, vaginal dryness, memory problems, insomnia, weight gain, anxiety, depression, fatigue and gastrointestinal problems can be caused by hormonal imbalance, and that solutions are available!

Koldtec
Koldtec.com

Koldtec is the world's coldest cooling towel. It's made in Canada of sustainable bamboo with engineered ice inside. The fabric is lightweight and absorbent, and in a wide range of colour options. Used by athletes and yoga enthusiasts, travellers and women navigating hot flashes. Wear at home, work or keep on your nightstand for instant relief from night sweats. Designed to direct instant cooling to the pulse points in your neck. Travel tube included keeps towel chilled for up to three hours.

Cathy McCann, CNTP
Nutrition Therapy Practitioner & Life Coach
McCannNutrition.com

I practice personalized nutrition therapy—targeting your unique issues with whole foods and high quality supplements. I don't advocate "diets." I believe in healthy living and making lifestyle changes that develop into habits. As a life coach, I support you to identify your goals and the obstacles that are keeping you from reaching them. Nutrition and life coaching work together to support women in midlife to nourish their bodies AND souls, heal years of neglect, and thrive in their exciting second half.

Jill Prescott
Spiritual Badass
JillPrescott.ca

We asked: What is the one thing you want women to know about perimenopause? **Jill said:** Welcome sister, to your life! Now is the time for celebration, for you have arrived at the place of wisdom. The preparation that has been your life until now is complete. All that is left for you to do is love. Do so with utter abandon, giving zero fucks about what the uninitiated think!

Leila Sahabi, ND
Naturopathic Doctor
DrLeilaSahabi.com

Dr. Leila Sahabi is dedicated to enhancing the health and quality of life for her patients by providing a comprehensive array of natural therapies. Her naturopathic medical practice is focused on the treatment of female hormonal imbalances, gastrointestinal conditions, autoimmune conditions, skin disorders and heavy metal toxicity. Dr. Sahabi utilizes various therapies including: bioidentical hormone replacement therapy, chelation therapy, nutritional intravenous therapy, homeopathy and dietary counselling.

For a more extensive list of resources, please visit
MenopauseChicks.com/find-an-expert

Author Biography

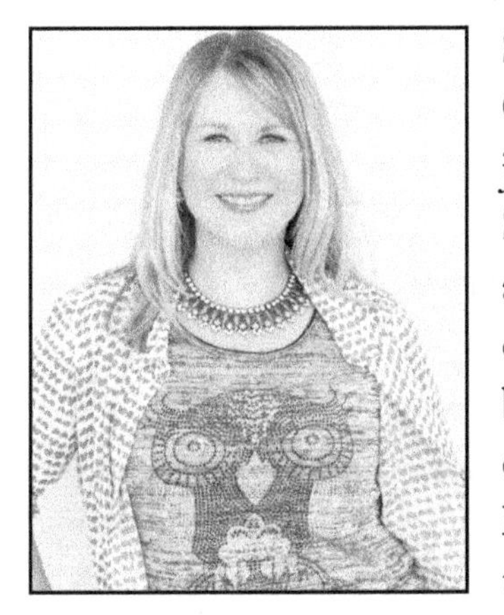

Shirley introduces herself as a Menopause Chick. Now 51, her perimenopause journey began more than ten years ago. Sore boobs, sleep deprivation, depression and brain fog led Shirley to her doctor's office, the book store and "Dr. Google," but she was left feeling confused, overwhelmed and alone. At 46, she launched MenopauseChicks.com onto the world stage to empower women to talk openly about perimenopause and menopause, to navigate midlife health information and to connect to women's health professionals.

Since that time, Shirley spoke at TEDxGastownWomen, Pecha Kucha, received a *YWCA Vancouver Woman of Distinction Award* and Menopause Chicks has been featured in the National Post, Toronto Star, and OWN (Oprah Winfrey Network). In April 2016, Shirley hosted the first-ever online menopause party celebrating her own menopause milestone. She and rock star, Bif Naked, discussed learning to love menopause, while women tuned in to share their stories in a private online community.

That private online community now fields an average of 15,000 questions and comments every month. Members regard the group as unbiased, trustworthy and the "go-to" place to get their questions answered and to affirm they are not alone.

Shirley's marketing & communications career spans 30 years, she holds a certificate in Peer Counselling from the University of British Columbia, and she is mom to two teenagers and one golden doodle.

Let's keep the conversation going

Private Online Community:	Facebook.com/groups/MenopauseChicks
Facebook:	Facebook.com/MenopauseChicks
Twitter:	@MenopauseChicks
Instagram:	@MenopauseChicks & @MOKITAforMIDLIFE
Email:	shirley@MenopauseChicks.com
TEDx Talk:	Tinyurl.com/ShirleyWeirTedTalk
Websites:	MenopauseChicks.com MOKITALive.com

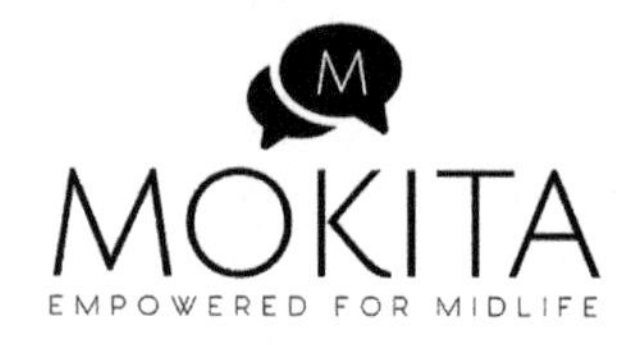

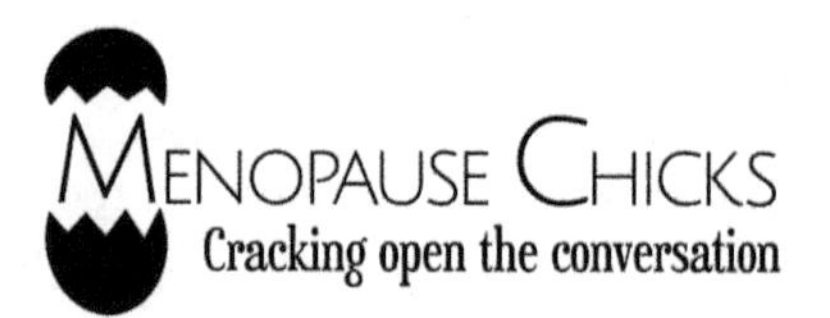

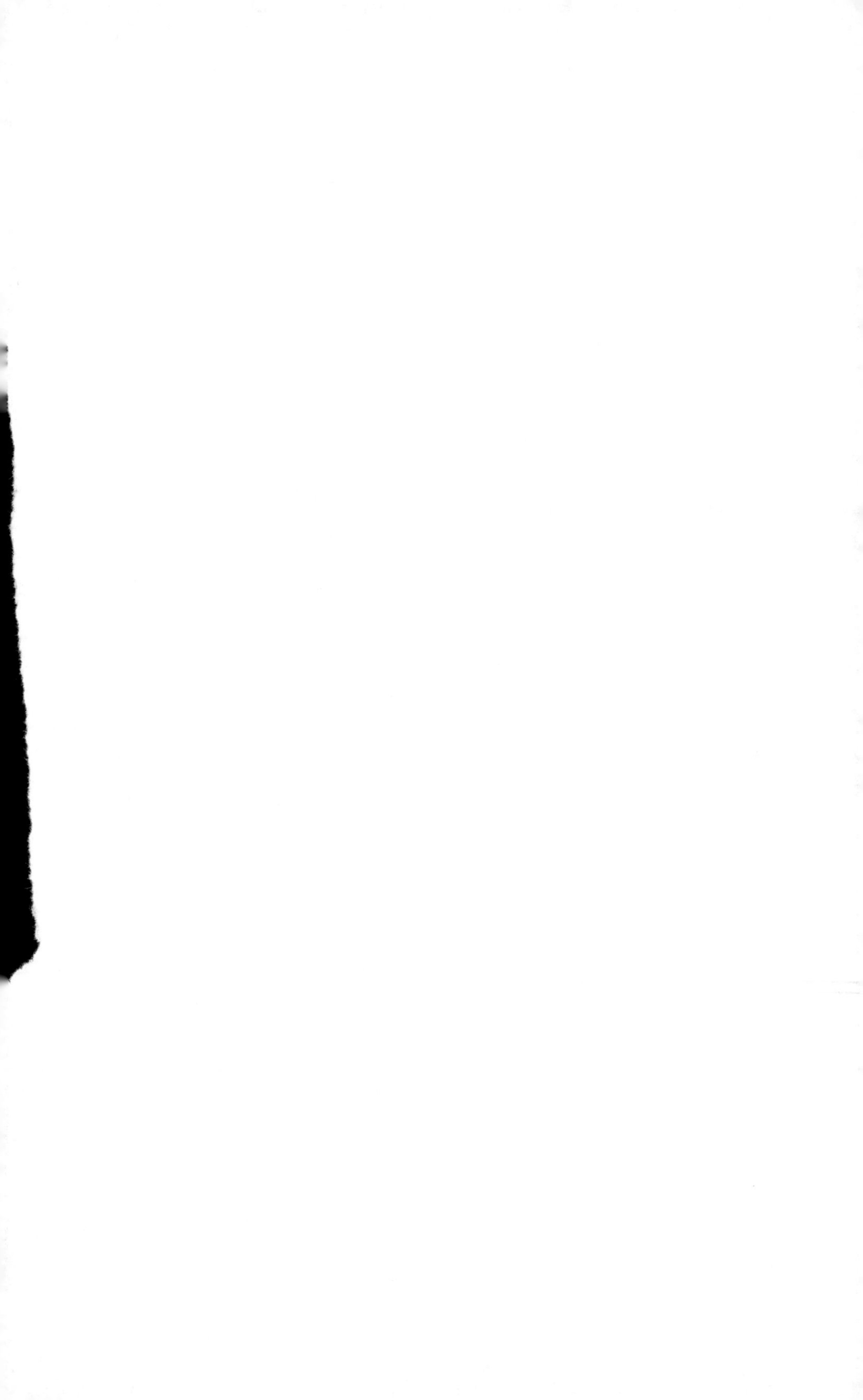

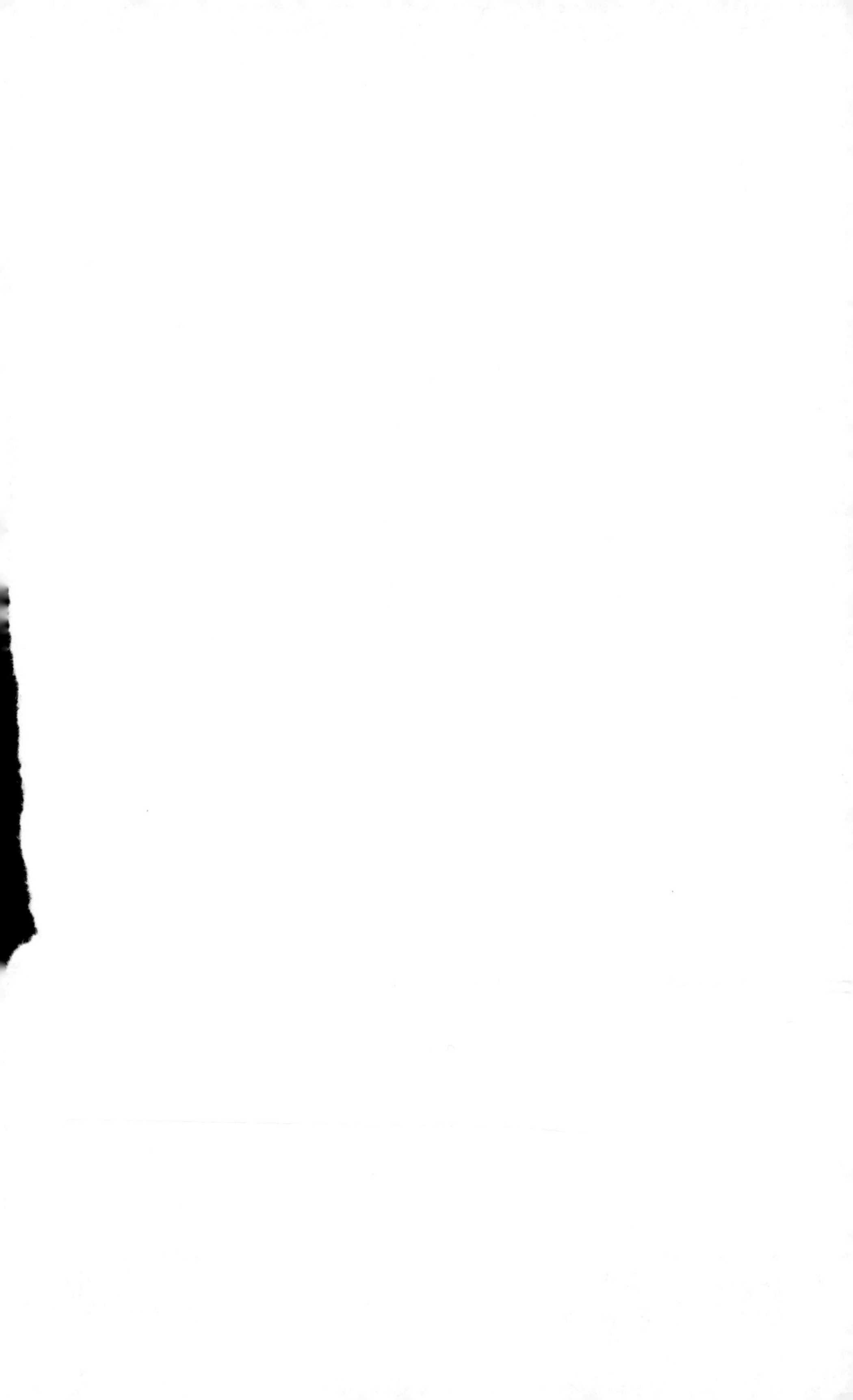

CPSIA information can be obtained
at www.ICGtesting.com
Printed in the USA
LVHW021658140419
614080LV00005B/121/P

9 781999 470104